## Special Praise for *Everyday Narcissism*

"This book gives us a new and very helpful way to look
at narcissism. It reminds us of truths we already knew
or suspected but have discounted or forgotten. *Everyday
Narcissism* is an easy read, and it is filled with help, good will,
and hope. I am wildly enthusiastic about the book!"

**Jean Illsley Clark**
Bestselling author of *Self-Esteem: A Family Affair,
Growing Up Again,* and *How Much Is Too Much?*

"*Everyday Narcissism* unfolds a way to understand why we
are the way we are and do what we do in relationships,
even if it's not good for us. Nancy Van Dyken exposes five
erroneous myths about a common perception that our needs
will be met if we meet the needs of others first. She helps us
understand what gives rise to these myths and offers lots of
ways to address them, much to our benefit."

**Connie Dawson**
Coauthor of *Growing Up Again*

"*Everyday Narcissism* is a spirited book that's filled with useful
insights and self-help suggestions. Nancy Van Dyken turns the
growing problem of narcissism around by helping us look at
ourselves, rather than judging everyone else. Her Five Myths,
Feelings Lists, Needs List, and many easy activities focus the
reader on practical steps anyone can take. By making it simple,
Van Dyken helps us nurture ourselves while also paying better
attention to our relationships."

**Bill Eddy**
Coauthor of *Splitting*

T0163986

"This little book offers its readers a BIG liberation! Wisely and sensitively crafted, Nancy Van Dyken examines EN—everyday narcissism—in an informed, honest, and nonjudgmental voice. This is a hopeful, positive gem of a book that I could not put down. I, for one, benefitted from its insights and am putting into practice its many lessons."

**Scherrie A. Foster**
Professor of Communication, Fond du Lac Tribal
and Community College

# EVERYDAY NARCISSISM

# EVERYDAY NARCISSISM

## *Yours, Mine, and Ours*

NANCY VAN DYKEN

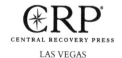

CENTRAL RECOVERY PRESS

LAS VEGAS

Central Recovery Press (CRP) is committed to publishing exceptional materials addressing addiction treatment, recovery, and behavioral healthcare topics.

For more information, visit www.centralrecoverypress.com.

Publisher:   Central Recovery Press
             3321 N. Buffalo Drive
             Las Vegas, NV 89129


22 21 20 19 18 17    1 2 3 4 5

Library of Congress Cataloging-in-Publication Data

Names: Van Dyken, Nancy, author.
Title: Everyday narcissism : yours, mine, and ours / Nancy Van Dyken ;
   foreword by Anne Katherine.
Description: Las Vegas : Central Recovery Press, 2017.
Identifiers: LCCN 2017012630 (print) | LCCN 2017025417 (ebook) | ISBN
   9781942094463 (ebook) | ISBN 9781942094456 (paperback)
Subjects: LCSH: Narcissism. | Self-actualization (Psychology) | Interpersonal
   relations. | BISAC: HEALTH & FITNESS / Healthy Living. | PSYCHOLOGY /
   Interpersonal Relations. | SELF-HELP / Personal Growth / Self-Esteem.
Classification: LCC BF575.N35 (ebook) | LCC BF575.N35 V36 2017 (print) | DDC
   155.2/32--dc23
LC record available at https://lccn.loc.gov/2017012630

Photo of Nancy Van Dyken by Peter Van Dyken. Used with permission.

**Publisher's Note:** This book contains general information about behavioral healthcare matters and related issues. The information is not medical advice. This book is not an alternative to medical advice from your doctor or other professional healthcare provider.

Our books represent the experiences and opinions of their authors only. Every effort has been made to ensure that events, institutions, and statistics presented in our books as facts are accurate and up-to-date. To protect their privacy, the names of some of the people, places, and institutions in this book may have been changed.

*Cover design by The Book Designers. Interior design by Sara Streifel, Think Creative Design.*

I dedicate this book to my grandchildren, Sierra Jane and Juniper Mae, who teach me how to be with them without giving them everyday narcissism messages and how to explore their world without the constraints of everyday narcissism. You continue to teach me the joy of living and how to love with a totally open heart.

And to Kelsey Jane, my daughter, who, because of my deep love for her, continually inspires me to be a better person and mother.

## The Five Myths of Everyday Narcissism

1. We are responsible for—and have the power to control—how other people feel and behave.

2. Other people are responsible for—and have the power to control—the way we feel and behave.

3. The needs and wants of other people are more important than our own.

4. Following the rules is also more important than addressing our needs and feelings.

5. We are not lovable as we are; we can only become lovable through what we do and say.

# Table of Contents

## Healing Activities

## Healing Tools

# Author's Note

Most of the stories in this book are either true or based on living people and actual situations. However, I have changed names and details to protect people's privacy. In a small number of cases, I have created composite characters based on multiple living people. In a few other cases—Isabel and her son Sam, for instance—each story is a hypothetical illustration of a key point. The fictional origins of such stories will be clear in context.

# Acknowledgments

I would like to acknowledge and thank my greatest teacher and lesson giver, my daughter Kelsey. As I made mistakes in my own parenting, my love for her kept me looking inward, seeking my own healing to improve my parenting. It is here that I discovered my own narcissism— how I'd been hurt by narcissism and how I had unintentionally hurt my lovely daughter with it as well.

I wish to thank my clients, who elected to trust me and believe that I could help them on their healing journeys. I am grateful for their willingness to walk into their own wounds and emotions, their strength in sharing them with me, and their courage to change.

I want to thank my first editor, Scott Edelstein, who was able to work magic with what I wrote. I appreciate his undying belief in the importance of this book; his confidence that I had something important to share; his continuous challenges to have me think things through and explore key topics more thoroughly; and his help in getting clear about what I was trying to say. He did all this with kindness, gentleness, acceptance, and encouragement. Scott, I am deeply grateful.

My thanks to everyone at Central Recovery Press—especially Valerie Killeen, Eliza Tutellier, and Patrick Hughes—who helped this book become everything I hoped it would be.

And to my family and friends who never left my side as I struggled with my ideas and my weariness of writing; all of you consistently believed that what I was doing mattered. Thank you.

"Happiness is when what you think,
what you say, and what you do
are in harmony."

*Mohandas Gandhi*

"In the long run, we shape our lives,
and we shape ourselves. The process
never ends until we die. And the
choices we make are ultimately
our own responsibility."

*Eleanor Roosevelt*

# FOREWORD

## Finding Your Way Back

Carrying the well-being of others on your own shoulders? Heavy, isn't it?

Meanwhile a very important life is being neglected. Yours.

We humans take extraordinary measures to feel safe, even sacrificing awareness of our truest selves in order to follow explicit and implicit rules. On that path, we can stray so far from our authentic center that we don't know that we've lost ourselves. Our own false self then relates to the false selves of others. How precarious is that?

My cat can't read. Even if I could bear to punish or withdraw from him, or if I used all my best skills to teach him, he still would be unable to read. (And imagine how our relationship would be affected, were I to continue to pressure him to live up to my expectations.)

Yet well-meaning parents routinely try to enforce behavior that is beyond a child's normal developmental capacity.

What do you imagine this does to a child? What did it do to you, when you were expected to handle a feeling or task that you weren't old enough for? How did your parents handle it, when you couldn't?

And if you're a parent, how can you avoid passing on the same downward spiral of internal neglect? How can you avoid demanding the impossible of others, especially after years of being immersed in myths yourself?

Forced compliance with cultural myths that are contrary to internal integrity, and even common sense, inevitably sets up problems with authority.

We all have a relationship with authority. We can struggle with it every day our whole lives and not be aware of the energy it uses or the cost of the struggle. This struggle can take many forms—love/hate, insist/resist, open compliance hiding secret defiance, open defiance leading to self-sabotage, overt or subtle domination, and/or passive resistance.

We may reward and please others, while simultaneously digging out the ground they are standing on. We can even force ourselves into internal compliance, while losing all awareness of honest reactions. We learn to wear a mask so smoothly that the edges of the mask graft to our skin.

What is your relationship with authority? Is yours healthy and sensible, or an ongoing struggle—at work or in professional situations, in your intimate relationships, and within yourself?

Do you defy your own needs or leanings? Shush inner guidance? Force unreasonable control over natural processes? And does your body resist you, or manifest the resulting tension by attacking itself? Are you sometimes surprised by sudden and impulsive explosions of anger?

Beneath this struggle is your own weeping self.

Through this thoughtful book, you will discover your own automatic behaviors that consume your time and energy. You will track their origins and then free yourself from them. You will uncover attitudes and thoughts that were programmed into you when you were just a tot, and your brain was still being formed, and replace them with messages that are more loving, honest, and effective.

With *Everyday Narcissism*, you can find your way back.

You will unearth the myths that have sidetracked your life, and reinstate boundaries that help you heal rather than suffer. You will channel yourself toward the life that belongs to you—a life that you create as you discover your own truest focus and deepest resources.

You will emancipate honest feelings that have been trapped in vaults deep inside you. By lifting out of darkness those closeted parts of yourself, you will discover a fuller self, release your own wisdom, and free energy that can fuel travel in your own best direction.

Do you know where that direction goes? Maybe not. And you need not fear your deepest self.

Even if you suspect that a fiery layer of anger lies dormant, you need not fear your deepest self. That anger is like a battery. It is stored energy. As with any energy source, learning how to handle it will empower you.

*Everyday Narcissism* will raise your awareness of your own layers. It will also give you tools to gently bring those layers into the light, according to your own best timing.

You have the potential to emerge from your cocoon of inauthenticity, to find a peaceful internal grace as you tune into your own profound self-authority that can orchestrate your unique best life.

**Anne Katherine**

Bestselling author of *Boundaries*
and *Where to Draw the Line*

1

# The Myths

"Live outside your comfort zone;
there are great discoveries there."

*Caroline Aron*

Narcissism is a belief that the world revolves around us, and that what happens in the world happens because of us. This belief is as common, and as pervasive, as it is erroneous.

Most of us live with a garden-variety form of narcissism that's so embedded we don't even know we have it. As a result, we suffer deeply and unnecessarily.

I call this *everyday narcissism*, or EN.

Nearly all of us are everyday narcissists—you, me, our friends, our children, our parents, our other relatives, our coworkers, our partners, and our neighbors. This narcissism comes from a combination of childhood wounds and enduring myths we were taught at a very young age. The more emotionally wounded we are, and the more we buy into these myths, the more narcissistic we tend to become.

These powerful myths get ingrained into our thinking, and we believe them because people we love and trust—our parents—initially teach them to us, while other adults in our lives regularly reinforce them. Let's begin by looking at the first four of these myths. (We'll examine the fifth myth in the following chapter.)

## Myth 1: We Are Responsible for—and Have the Power to Control—How Other People Feel and Behave

When we live our lives according to this first myth, we are in a constant state of hypervigilance, fearing that we won't belong or fit in if we don't make others happy through what we do and say. We spend much of our time trying to figure out what other people want, what they need, and what will make them happy.

Meanwhile, we consistently ignore ourselves—what *we* want, what *we* need, and what will make *us* happy. We neglect ourselves, believing that if others are happy with us, they will love us—and, as a result, we will become happy, too. We may also take credit for other people's happiness, as if it occurred because we performed so well.

When we believe this, we constantly watch how others react to us. If they are unhappy, we assume it is because we did something wrong. We tell ourselves that if only we had said or done or been something different, they would be happy. We assume we've failed and we feel ashamed or burdened or unlovable. Thus we live in fear of rejection and disapproval.

Honesty takes a back seat to pleasing each other when more or less everyone lives according to this myth. Worse, over time, each of us loses our sense of who we are. We no longer know ourselves; we only know what others want.

We imagine that making others happy will bring us happiness. Yet if we live a life of pleasing others and avoiding conflict, of consistently doing things for others at our own expense, we are not happy at all—because without honesty there can be no intimacy, no connection, and no genuine love.

## Myth 2: Other People Are Responsible for—and Have the Power to Control—the Way We Feel and Behave

### ANGELINE AND GARY

Like most of us, Angeline has been raised to believe Myths 1 and 2. As a result, when her nine-year-old son Gary does something that bothers her, she says to him, "You've made me angry at you."

Instead of focusing on Gary's actions—for example, he didn't put away his toys, as he promised he'd do—she makes the problem the *way she feels* about his actions. Instead of Gary learning that he is responsible for taking care of his possessions, he learns that he is responsible for fixing his mother's feelings.

In an extreme version of Myth 2, a parent blames their child for the parent's feelings—*and* for how the parent *responds* to those feelings. "Now look what you've done. You make me so upset that I dropped my tea mug and broke it." Or, "If you had cleaned up your room like you promised, I wouldn't have gotten so angry and yelled at you."

When people in a relationship believe Myth 2, their disagreements typically turn into ever-escalating arguments, and no satisfactory resolution is ever found. Each person holds the other responsible for their own happiness or satisfaction and blames the other for not providing it. Each then resents the other for not doing their part.

## Myth 3: The Needs and Wants of Other People Are More Important than Our Own

This third myth implies that our own needs and wants don't really matter, and it is especially pervasive for children. Thus Myth 3 naturally erodes our self-esteem and self-confidence.

Myths 1 and 3 are typically taught together, so they reinforce one another. As we learn that we're responsible for how others feel, we also learn that other people matter far more than we do—or that we don't matter at all.

## Myth 4: Following the Rules Is Also More Important than Addressing Our Needs and Feelings

When rules are properly designed and applied, they can help remove chaos from our lives. This is why we have stoplights and stop signs. However, when rules are made more important than the human beings they are meant to serve, people become wounded—especially if they are young.

One of the hallmarks of EN is that it often puts rules before people by elevating obedience and compliance and discounting genuine human needs. Teaching children to not interrupt adult conversations is important. However, they also need to be able to interrupt if there is an emergency.

## Adding Up the Myths

These four myths don't just pervade our culture; they are cultural norms. We teach them to our kids to help them grow up and become functional adults. Some people would even say the myths of EN help children learn to be kind and thoughtful.

However, the myths of EN do nothing of the sort. They make all of us—those who learn it and those who teach it—smaller, younger, less functional, and more wounded.

To teach kindness to others, we must first be kind ourselves. EN, and the myths that support and perpetuate it, are not kind.

Yet these myths are everywhere. As we age, our mentors, teachers, and role models—and, eventually, our peers—all live by these four myths and teach them to us.

Year after year, we repeat these myths to ourselves and learn to act them out, over and over. With each thought and each action, we internally reinforce their hold on us. Eventually we come to believe them and live by them. Then we also teach them to others.

By the time we are adolescents, most of us have internalized all four myths—and we have put them together into the following narrative, which we constantly, yet subtly, communicate to each other:

- When you feel angry, sad, or hurt, or when you act in ways I don't like, I am responsible for your feelings and behavior. This means it's my responsibility to fix you or the situation, so that you feel better and act appropriately.

- And when you feel good or act in ways I like, it's because I did the right thing.

- Furthermore, when I feel bad, it's your fault—and your responsibility to fix me or the situation so I feel better.

This narrative is the basis for the everyday narcissism that almost everyone shares.

Why is this a form of narcissism? Because, as a result of the lifelong training I've just described, almost all of us live by the following unconscious (and false) principles:

- I am responsible for how other people feel and behave. Therefore, I experience myself as all-powerful.

- I am responsible for how others act toward *me*. Therefore, I once again experience myself as all-powerful.

- Other people are responsible for how *I* feel and behave— and are supposed to make me feel safe, happy, and okay. Therefore, I am the center of the universe.

> The myths and principles of EN take root
> in our psyches because they are taught to us,
> over and over, by people we trust.

The first two principles of EN involve an unrealistic obligation *to* others (and their unrealistic expectations of us). The third involves our own unrealistic expectations *of* others.

The myths and principles of EN take root in our psyches because they are taught to us, over and over, by people we trust. Yet the myths and principles wound us deeply.

Worse, in our mostly misguided efforts to soothe our wounds, we often wound others in much the same ways that we were wounded. We then pass on our everyday narcissism to others, as if it were a virus.

## Outgrowing Narcissism

In order to survive, babies or young children need the world to revolve around them. Parents must attend to them closely, meeting their needs and keeping them safe.

As we grow older, however, we naturally want to become ever more independent. By age two, we start letting our parents know that we can do things ourselves, such as put on our coats and take off our shoes. With each passing year, our parents back off a little further, and we are quick to remind them that this is what we want and expect of them.

By nature, as we grow older and gain more skills and confidence, we would outgrow our childhood narcissism. Over time, systematically, we would seek more and more independence. We would stop demanding or expecting the world to revolve around us. We would learn to do more and more things ourselves: tie our shoes, ride a bike, comb our hair, brush our teeth, and so on. We gain our physical independence slowly and methodically.

However, our process of emotional independence is thwarted. Even as we gain more physical independence, we simultaneously internalize the EN myths and the principles that accompany them, and we develop emotional dependence rather than independence. We believe, in all the perverse ways I previously described, that the world *does* revolve around us.

As we mature, most of us learn to meet our own physical needs. Emotionally, however, most of us struggle with everyday narcissism, which stifles our emotional development and our independence. We carry this EN into adulthood and into most or all of our relationships.

Nearly all of us suffer from EN without knowing it. It has a tremendous impact on our lives, creating anxiety, anger, depression, an unnatural emotional dependence on others, and less fulfilling relationships.

## The Role of Trauma

Trauma is always felt deeply—and remembered—by our body. To the body, trauma is invariably experienced as an assault, whether physical, emotional, verbal, psychological, sexual, or spiritual.

When most of us think of trauma, we think of extremely painful events such as incest, abuse, rape, war, assault, serious injury, severe betrayal, extreme neglect, or great and unexpected loss. However, trauma can also result from small, painful incidents that get repeated many times. This is often the case with the everyday narcissism most of us are exposed to as children.

EN can be seen as a form of neglect, in which a child's emotional (and sometimes physical) needs are ignored in favor of those of adults. Through EN, day after day and year after year, most of us experienced a slow, repetitive grinding down of our self-worth, self-confidence, and self-trust.

### CASSIE AND HER GRANDMOTHER

Four-year-old girl Cassie is told by her mother to give Grandma a kiss goodbye. Cassie doesn't want to because Grandma just hurt her feelings. Nevertheless, her mother insists—with annoyance in her voice—and tells her, "If you don't kiss Grandma, she'll be hurt.'"

This is a classic and common example of how we teach our kids Myths 1 and 3. Although Cassie is only four, she is taught that she is responsible for how Grandma feels—and how Grandma feels is important, while how Cassie feels is not.

Cassie's mom is trying to teach her something important: to be sensitive to others' feelings. However, what Cassie is actually beginning to learn is to be sensitive to others' feelings *and to ignore her own.*

Because of the incident, Cassie hurts. She doesn't have a terrible wound, of course; it's more like a paper cut.

> However, when this same lesson is repeated over and over, in many different contexts, it becomes a damaging wound.
>
> I call this *hazy trauma*. It's not the result of a single big event. It's the cumulative effect of many emotional paper cuts. It's also a form of neglect because Cassie's own feelings get repeatedly ignored, discounted, or pushed aside.

As psychologist Patrick Carnes has noted, neglect can be harder to recover from than incest or physical abuse—precisely because there is no single big, causal incident. Instead, the trauma is hazy and hard to clearly identify because it is made up of many smaller, recurring events. And, in the case of EN, *these events are seen as normal (or even instructive and beneficial) by most adults*, whereas incest and physical abuse are not—and, indeed, are against the law.

Our normal response to trauma has several aspects. First, our body experiences fear in the limbic part of our brain. When this occurs, the amygdala (within the limbic system) kicks in, creating a fight, flight, or freeze response. At the same time, our left prefrontal cortex—the thinking, organizing, sequencing, and impulse controlling part of our brain—shuts off. Our survival instincts and emotions are now in charge. Rational thinking is literally not available to us because the rational part of our brain has been temporarily unplugged (or, as some therapists say, *overruled* or *hijacked*).

This is why, when we see that our kitchen curtains are on fire, we automatically start moving toward safety. We don't sit still and thoughtfully analyze the cause of the fire or what possessions to save.

Trauma may also impact other parts of our brain. As a result, we may have little or no conscious memory of the cause of the trauma, especially if it occurred in preverbal childhood, when we didn't have words to remember or explain our experience.

Usually, though, our body remembers the sights, sounds, tastes, smells, or other sensory information associated with any trauma. When we later experience a similar sight or sound or taste, our body may automatically get triggered and shift into a trauma response. Suddenly, we will feel or act as if the original trauma is happening *right now*, in the present moment.

> ... intense and abrupt emotional reactions
> are usually trauma responses from an old
> wound that just got triggered.

Our body never forgets. It continues to react to those triggers, whenever and wherever they appear, until the trauma is healed. A classic case is the war veteran who, while playing with his kids in his own backyard, hears a car backfire. Because the sound reminds his body of a gunshot, fear kicks in, and his amygdala takes over. Without thinking, he dives for cover. As we will see, the trauma of everyday narcissism has similar effects on most of us when we re-experience—or are reminded of—painful sights, sounds, smells, and feelings from our childhood.

Have you ever had a sudden, strong emotional reaction to a seemingly small incident, comment, or gesture? You yourself may have been surprised by the intensity of your reaction. These intense and abrupt emotional reactions are usually trauma responses from an old wound that just got triggered—the result of the EN we were taught as children.

## The Takeaway

This book will help you understand how everyday narcissism manifests in your own life, and it will teach you to recognize it *and heal it*.

As a result, you will grow into a life of greater happiness; more fulfilling relationships; less reactivity; greater responsiveness to the people and things that matter to you; and more meaning. You'll also learn to recognize everyday narcissism in others and respond to their EN in healthy ways. Best of all, you will begin to understand your life in a whole new way. You will learn to recognize more choices and greater freedom in your life. You will begin to relax and enjoy your life more. You will rediscover your true self and live a life of greater joy.

# 2

# Everyday Narcissism vs. Clinical Narcissism

"When the healthy pursuit of self-interest
and self-realization turns into self-absorption,
other people can lose their intrinsic value in
our eyes and become mere means to the
fulfillment of our needs and desires."

*P.M. Forni*

It's important to understand the difference between everyday narcissism and what is often called *clinical narcissism*.

Clinical narcissism, technically known as *narcissistic personality disorder*, is a diagnosable mental illness, one of ten types of personality disorders. The Mayo Clinic offers the following definition of a personality disorder:

A personality disorder is a type of mental disorder in which you have a rigid and unhealthy pattern of thinking, functioning, and behaving. A person with a personality disorder has trouble perceiving and relating to situations and to people. This causes significant problems and limitations in relationships, social encounters, work, and school.

Personality disorders are divided into three groups: *anxious*, *suspicious*, and *emotional/impulsive*. Clinical narcissism is an emotional/impulsive personality disorder.

Everyday narcissism, however, is *not* a personality disorder—and not something that can be diagnosed by a therapist. It's a familiar outcome of being raised by less-than-perfect parents in a less-than-Utopian society. It's not healthy, yet it's extremely common.

In recent years, the words *narcissism* and *narcissistic* have become widely used in everyday conversation. In that context, they usually refer to someone who is extremely self-involved and doesn't care about anyone else. People often use the term to refer to a boss, coworker, family member, partner, or neighbor.

This informal adaptation of a clinical term roughly parallels the use of the word *depressed*. A lot of people use that word when they temporarily feel sadness, hopelessness, or despair. This is a very different state from someone who suffers from clinical depression, which is a serious, sometimes chronic, and sometimes life-threatening disorder. Something similar happened in the 1980s and 1990s, when generous, cooperative people were occasionally labeled *codependent* in everyday conversation.

Let's dig a bit deeper into clinical narcissism.

People with narcissistic personality disorder have a constant and overwhelming need for attention—and, usually, for admiration, praise, and validation. At a social gathering, they dominate the conversation. At work, they seek the highest possible position and regularly insist their ideas are the best.

Clinical narcissists typically exaggerate their accomplishments and talents—and genuinely believe those exaggerations. They lie often, blatantly, and shamelessly. They have a greatly overblown sense of their own importance and often come across as extremely arrogant.

They tend to be bossy, judgmental, perfectionistic, controlling, and power-hungry. They have no qualms about exploiting, cheating—or, in some cases, destroying—other people to get what they want.

## GEORGIA

Georgia lies in a hospital bed, only days away from death. Her daughter Clara sits besides her, holding her hand; her dog Brownie relaxes at the foot of her bed.

Georgia says to her daughter, "Have you made all the arrangements for my cremation and burial?"

Clara nods and squeezes her mother's hand. "It's all taken care of, Mom."

"One other thing," Georgia says. "I want Brownie cremated and buried with me."

Clara pulls her hand away. "Brownie's still young and healthy. He'll probably live another six or seven years."

"No. I love Brownie as much as any human being possibly can. I want him cremated, and then I want you to mix his ashes with mine."

Georgia's wishes are *not* a reflection of everyday narcissism. They are symptoms of narcissistic personality disorder, a serious mental disorder.

People with narcissistic personality disorder have a strong need to be right in every situation. They genuinely believe they know and understand everything, and that they are never wrong. They also become aggressive when anyone challenges them.

This book is not about people with narcissistic personality disorder. It's about you and me.

Most clinical narcissists have a strong sense of entitlement. They feel they are owed constant adulation, attention, and praise. They also feel they deserve to always get their way. Yet they have little or no insight into themselves, and they are utterly unable to empathize with someone else or see a situation from their viewpoint.

Perhaps most notably, people with narcissistic personality disorder don't realize there's anything wrong with them. In fact, they think that everything about themselves is just right—and better than everyone else.

This book is *not* about people with narcissistic personality disorder. It's about you and me—and our relatives, partners, coworkers, neighbors, and friends. It's about a form of emotional wounding that is as common as headaches and sore throats, yet far more painful and damaging. Most of all, it's about healing the wounds of your own everyday narcissism and creating the life you truly long for.

# 3

# How It Begins

"I was always looking outside myself for
strength and confidence, but it comes from
within. It is there all the time."

*Anna Freud*

We're all born narcissistic. This is a good thing. When we're very small, the world is *supposed* to revolve around us and our physical, psychological, and emotional needs. Up until about age two, a child *needs* to be the center of their parents' world.

If, as kids, our needs are regularly met year after year, we feel physically safe and unconditionally loved and confident. When we reach adulthood, we are physically and emotionally ready for the world and free of any EN. Yet this is generally not what children experience. Instead, most of us grow up emotionally wounded. Our psyches are bathed in EN, and we are surrounded by people who also suffer from EN.

As children, we each have a host of physical, spiritual, and emotional needs. These range from food, shelter, clothing, and safety to feeling counted, heard, believed, comforted, and valued. When we're young, we are wounded each time one of our physical and emotional needs is not met. As children, most of us are wounded often in this way.

Please note that I'm talking about needs, not wants. As children, we may *want* to go swimming; however, we *need* to be fed. Not always getting what we want—and learning to handle the disappointment we feel in response—are important parts of growing up. However, being dismissed or discounted or ignored *does* wound us.

Many of these wounds are both commonplace and invisible to adults. For example, a first grader tells her mother that she wants to wear her hair in braids. However, her mother insists that she wear a ponytail. A third grader wants to play soccer, while his father, who played baseball, insists that his son do the same. In both cases, the children don't feel heard, counted, or valued.

Parents are generally unaware of how and when they inflict these wounds. They are simply repeating the patterns they experienced when they were younger.

To help you see how commonplace these wounds are, and how small we are when they begin to affect us, let's look at two more detailed examples.

## BOBBY AND HIS FATHER

Bobby's parents, Ned and Michele, are getting him ready for a party for his first birthday. Both his parents are excited. Bobby doesn't understand much of what is going on, yet he sees there is a cake in the shape of a car, and he likes cake. People are hanging decorations, and his father is dressing him in a special outfit.

Soon his relatives start to arrive, and everyone starts to make a fuss over him. At first Bobby enjoys this. Then more and more people arrive. The house gets louder and louder and more and more crowded.

Bobby starts to feel uneasy and a little frightened by all the commotion and attention. He starts to cry. He looks around and sees his grandfather, whom he adores. He points to his grandfather and says, "I want to go to Grandpa!"

Bobby's father Ned is disappointed and upset. He and Michele planned this party for weeks. He is excited to present his son to the crowd and show everyone how great Bobby is. Now his son doesn't even want to be with him and wants to be with his grandpa instead. Plus, Bobby's crying is interrupting Ned's plans to show him off.

Ned tells his son, "Settle down, Bobby. Everything is okay. You're fine. It's a party. We're all here to have fun."

Yet Bobby doesn't feel that everything is fine. He insists on what *he* wants, what will help him feel good: being with Grandpa.

Begrudgingly, because he is feeling the pressure of Myth 2, Ned hands his son to Grandpa. Bobby feels his father's disapproval. He knows he's not doing what he is supposed to do: please his father (and follow Myth 1).

Neither Bobby nor Ned can recall this incident today. Nevertheless, on that day Bobby began to learn a lesson that would be repeated many more times throughout his childhood: he is expected to stifle his own wants and needs (Myth 3) and, instead, take care of his father (Myth 1).

It's normal and healthy for Ned to be proud of his son and for Bobby's parents to throw him a party and want to show him off to the relatives. However, when Ned made it Bobby's job to make Ned proud and happy, this was Ned's EN at work.

Ned carried his own childhood wounds inside him. He was the oldest of four children raised by a divorced, single mother who worked two jobs and was often exhausted. As a result, Ned's needs routinely weren't met. This wasn't because his mother was unloving; she was simply overwhelmed. Ned grew up feeling that his own needs and desires often didn't count (Myth 3). Bobby's behavior triggered in Ned that old pain of not counting. In his annoyance and anger (Myth 2), Ned unwittingly passed on a bit of his EN to his son.

Ned and Michele are loving and reasonably functional parents. As with most of us, though, EN has become part of who they are, how they make their way in the world, and how they raise their son.

This one event won't harm Bobby that much. The problem is that similar events will occur over and over, year after year, and no one—not Ned, or Michele, or Bobby—will recognize how the myths, the principles, and the pain of EN are being passed on from one generation to the next.

## KYOKO, HER MOTHER, AND HER GRANDMOTHER

Two-year-old Kyoko and her mother Ayami are visiting Kyoko's grandmother Mika on a hot summer afternoon. While Kyoko is busy playing with a doll and her mom is in the bathroom, her grandma suddenly picks up Kyoko and hugs her tightly.

Kyoko doesn't want her play to be interrupted. She is also hot and sweaty and doesn't want to be hugged tightly by anyone right now. So she tries to push herself away. In response, her grandma holds her tighter and says, "You're so cute! You're a perfect little doll!"

Trying to escape, and angry at how her grandma is treating her, Kyoko grabs the string of pearls from around her grandmother's neck and pulls on them. The necklace breaks, sending pearls scattering everywhere.

Kyoko's grandmother sets her down on the sofa and says angrily, "Shame on you! Look what you've done!" (Myth 2)

Ayami enters the room a moment later, sees the pearls all over the floor, kneels to pick them up, and acts out Myth 1.

Mika says to her daughter, "You need to teach your little one some manners!"

Ayami looks up at her daughter and says, "Honey, you need to be more careful. Look at the mess you made." Here she expresses and reinforces Myth 2. Now both adults are holding a two-year-old responsible for their unhappiness. This helps to teach the child Myth 1.

Kyoko can barely speak in sentences, let alone articulate her needs. When her grandmother forced her into an unwanted hug, Kyoko responded in a very appropriate way for a two-year-old, by trying to separate her body from her grandmother's. She clearly and honestly expressed her emotions and desires.

Kyoko's grandmother ignores this and does only what *she* wants. Understandably, Kyoko feels angry—and expresses that anger. Wouldn't *you* feel angry if someone hugged you against your will?

Then Kyoko's grandmother tells her that *she* did something wrong and shameful. A few seconds later, her mother also reprimands Kyoko for doing the wrong thing. Yet no one cares to understand Kyoko's actions. (This is Myth 3 in action.)

Although she is too young to name or understand her own emotions, Kyoko feels judged, rejected, shamed, overlooked, and alone.

Mika and Ayami are not bad people. They both love Kyoko and they both love each other. Neither one wants to harm Kyoko. Yet they both send Kyoko powerful messages that begin to embed the following myths in her:

Myth 1: Kyoko is supposed to make her grandmother and mother happy—and in this incident, she has done the opposite.

Myth 3: Kyoko's needs and wants don't matter; only those of adults do.

At age two, Kyoko is unable to consciously process any of this. Nevertheless, she gets the message loud and clear: *No matter what Grandma does to me, if I do something she doesn't like, she'll be mad at me and not like me—and it will be my fault.*

Mika also chastises her daughter, Ayami, using Myth 2. In essence, she tells Ayami, "Your parenting made me unhappy."

---

One core purpose of this book is to help you recognize EN when you see it—in both yourself and others—so you are able to name it, heal from it, and grow out of it.

Most of us are clueless about the myriad ways in which EN negatively affects our lives. This is because we don't recognize or think through our everyday narcissism; it all usually occurs beneath the surface of our consciousness. As a result, we're often confused, disappointed, or angry—and mystified at the depth of hurt or anger or craziness we can sometimes feel over ostensibly small things.

One core purpose of this book is to help you recognize EN when you see it—in both yourself and others—so you are able to name it, heal from it, and grow out of it.

## Unpacking the Myths

The five myths—combined with our human need to belong, to be loved, to be liked, and to be part of community—form the foundation of EN. Let's dive more deeply into each of the myths.

## Myth 1: We Are Responsible for—and Have the Power to Control—How Other People Feel and Behave

Starting when we are young, we are taught that our biggest job—no matter what age we are—is to make our parents and other adults feel happy, proud, successful, adequate, important, loved, and so on. Our second biggest job is to prevent them from acting in ways that hurt us or are harmful or inappropriate in general.

The adults around us initially teach us Myth 1 by saying things such as:

- "Tell your aunt how much you like the lime-green sweater she gave you or she'll be hurt."
- "Go with your father or he'll be disappointed."
- "If you don't text him right back, he'll feel bad."
- "Mom will be upset if you don't come over."

In all of these statements, an adult is asking a child to take care of an adult. These phrases teach children that they are responsible for adults, when in fact it is supposed to be the other way around.

We do this partly to help children learn to be sensitive to the feelings and needs of others. Yet kids also need to learn to be aware of and sensitive to *their own* feelings and needs, so they can express and manage them in healthy ways. Unfortunately, many of us are not taught to be sensitive to ourselves; instead, we're taught Myth 3. In practice, sensitivity to others is best taught by modeling rather than words.

In her book *Prisoners of Childhood*, psychologist Alice Miller writes,

Children who fulfill their parents' conscious or unconscious wishes are "good," but if they ever refuse to do so or express wishes of their own that go against those of their parents, they are called egoistic or inconsiderate [e.g., thoughtless, rude, selfish, uncaring].[1] It usually does not occur to the parents that they might need and use the child to fulfill their own egoistic wishes.

Over time, we learn to internalize such messages, and eventually our EN becomes perpetually reinforced. By the time we're adolescents, most of us say similar things to ourselves, as well as to other people in our lives:

- "Don't go. I'll be so lonely without you."
- "I'm disappointed that you don't like the gifts I gave you."
- "I'm hurt that you're choosing not to join us at the party."

---

1    The bracketed words are mine, not Miller's.

We could say these are simple statements of fact, which state how we feel and what we want. In the EN-oriented world we have created, however, that is *not* how the statements are usually intended or heard. The message beneath all of them is, *It's your job to take care of me and make me feel good. The way to do that is to do what I want. You're the one with the power—and the responsibility—to make me happy. It all revolves around you.*

Here are some other common examples of how this gets played out:

- If we throw a party and all the guests have a good time, we assume it's because we were a great host.
- If our boss calls us to her office, we assume we have done something wrong.
- If a neighbor visits us and she's in a grumpy mood, we assume it's because of something we said or did in her presence the last time we saw her.
- If we're a therapist—and, yes, therapists do often struggle with their own EN—we mentally take credit for a client's improved confidence and focus, when in fact the client did the work.

## KELLY AND HER MOTHER

Thirteen-year-old Kelly looks carefully through her closet. She and her family are about to go to a rock concert where her aunt is performing, and she wants to look her best—and her coolest.

She finally chooses a blue leather skirt and a turtleneck sweater. She looks at herself in the mirror and is very pleased with her choice.

When she goes downstairs, her mother looks at her and frowns. She says, "Oh, Kelly, your orange plaid skirt and your orange blouse look *so* much cuter on you. I thought you'd be wearing that."

Kelly is hurt and angry. She likes what she is wearing and feels confident and comfortable in it. She's tired of always having to dress the way her mother wants. Yet she knows that if she doesn't change her clothes, her mother will be angry and start to pout. (Myth 1)

Kelly has had enough experience with her mom's pouting to know what will come after that. Dad will ask what's wrong, and Mom will say, "It's your daughter. She thinks it's too much to ask her to wear what I want her to wear." (Myth 3) Then Dad will be angry and agitated because he doesn't know how to deal with his wife's pouting.

Kelly doesn't want to have to face all of this—or, worse, be blamed for it. So she stomps upstairs and puts on the orange outfit, which she doesn't particularly like, and which, to her, seems completely wrong for a rock concert. In the process, she ends up following Myths 1 and 3 (as well as Myth 5, which we'll get to shortly).

Kelly's parents know she is angry. Yet they don't care, so long as she changes her clothes.

Now that Kelly is in her orange outfit, Mom is happy and relaxed. As a result, Dad is happy and relaxed, too.

All the way to the concert, Kelly sits in the back seat of the car, pouting and fuming. No one in the front seat cares. And why would they? Their needs are being met.

Here is the message Kelly's mother sends her, courtesy of her EN—a message that Kelly hears loudly and clearly: *You need to dress to please me, not yourself. And if you don't dress how I want you to, you'll hurt and disappoint me.* Kelly experiences this as rejection. This is a clothing-focused version of Myth 1.

Kelly learns not to stand up for herself as often as she would like to. She comes to believe that the normal results of taking a stand will be shame and rejection, so most of the time she just gives in. Eventually she may find herself struggling with depression.

## Myth 2: Other People Are Responsible for—and Have the Power to Control—the Way We Feel and Behave

When we were children, adults blamed us for their unhappiness and bad behavior. We then experienced their disapproval, anger, and rejection for our ostensible failure to make them happy.

Feeling hurt by the rejection and blame, we in turn learned to blamed those adults for making us feel so miserable. Eventually a vicious circle of blame was created. Myth 2 is the consequence of others not following Myth 1.

Blaming is learned through modeling. When we are children and adults routinely blame us for their dissatisfaction, we learn that this is what normal human beings do. So we start blaming others for our unhappiness as well. As adults, we naturally continue this pattern.

Since we are supposed to make other people happy, they, in turn, are supposed to make us happy. Thus we live according to Myth 2. We hold others accountable for what we do and how we feel. When we are unhappy or angry or disappointed or sad, we blame other people for making us feel that way. They did the wrong thing, or said the wrong words, or used a nasty tone, or refused to look at us while they talked, or didn't call us back quickly enough. *Our* unhappiness is *their* fault.

We experience this in restaurants, when the server isn't fast or attentive enough; on the highway, when the person in front of us doesn't yield or isn't going fast enough; at work, when our boss doesn't tell us what a great job we are doing; and at home, when our kids don't even look up from their laptops when we walk in after a long, hard day of work.

We do the very same thing when we feel happy or serene: we attribute that feeling to what someone else did. This is particularly common when we're dating. We give the other person credit for our excitement or happiness or delight—when, in fact, those feelings arose from our willingness to open up to and connect with someone else. We give credit to the mirror for the reflection we see in it.

Because of our EN, when others do what we want, we don't just feel happy or pleased; we feel important, valued, respected, cared for, counted, and appreciated. When they don't do what we want, we feel just the opposite.

> ... controlling (or attempting to control) others
> usually leads to misery, not happiness.

As a result, because of our EN, we come to believe that *getting other people to do what we want will create our happiness.* Yet decades of research into human happiness tell us that this is utterly false; controlling (or attempting to control) others usually leads to misery, not happiness.

Nevertheless, this is the very conviction that almost all of us live by. In our attempts to control others, we criticize them, analyze them, manipulate them, guilt or shame them, blame them, call them names, ignore them, swear at them, hit them—or flatter them, beg them, or bribe them with sweetness or compliance or sex or money or attention.

In relationships where each person holds the other responsible for their own happiness, a game of hot potato evolves. People take turns blaming each other for how they feel, sharing in detail what the other person did wrong. No one wants to hold the hot potato—that is, accept blame for the other person's discomfort—for very long. No one wants to get stuck being the villain. So the potato gets passed back and forth endlessly.

The most dangerous form of Myth 2 appears in violent relationships. Abusers tell their partners repeatedly that the abuse is the partner's fault. If only their partner would act right, speak right, cook supper right, not use the wrong tone of voice, cut the onions right, never be late, never forget the umbrella, etc., then the abuser would treat the partner well. They tell their partner the abuse is the result of the partner's bad behavior. The partner may believe this, too, because it is an expression of Myth 1.

Most of us even apply Myth 2 to inanimate objects. We expect our computers and phones and cars and zippers and plumbing to always work perfectly, and, because of our EN, we get mad at them when they don't. We curse our smartphones or yell at our computers, even though we know perfectly well that they're only devices. Yet because Myth 2 has become so deeply ingrained in us, we imagine that these objects are somehow responsible for—and have the power to control—the way we feel and behave. We imagine that it's their job to make us happy, rather than just perform a function.

## Myth 3: The Needs and Wants of Other People Are More Important than Our Own

Myth 3 is a natural consequence of Myth 1. If we must please others—and if we must focus on what *they* want and need and ignore our own wants and needs, or risk losing their love and support—what other conclusion can we possibly come to?

As we will see, the way to begin healing from Myth 3 is to look inward at what genuinely matters to us—what *we* want, need, and care about—and then act on it.

---

### CHAUNCEY, HIS FATHER, AND HIS MUSIC TEACHER

When he is in the sixth grade, Chauncey tells his father he wants to learn to play the trombone. Instead, his school's music teacher insists he first learn to play the French horn, a much more difficult instrument.

When Chauncey tells his father about this, his dad calls the teacher and says, "Why can't my son learn whatever instrument he wants to?" The music teacher says, "The school band doesn't have a single French horn player, and it already has two trombone players. If your son would learn the French horn, it would help out the whole school."

Chauncey's mother and father discuss the situation and decide that the music teacher's needs and wants—and those of the school band—are more important than Chauncey's.

They don't realize they're doing this, of course. Because of their EN, they want to look like cooperative people and please the band director. They don't understand how much they are discounting their son and teaching him Myth 3.

They tell their son of their decision and say, "Just try the French horn for a couple of years. Maybe you'll like it. If you still want to play the trombone by the time you're in eighth grade, we'll stand behind you."

Chauncey feels betrayed, then outraged, then despondent. The incident teaches him two things. First, to adults, his musical desires aren't important—only the adults' desires are. Second, adults often join together to outmaneuver or overpower kids.

Although Chauncey dutifully takes up the French horn, he is deeply wounded by the incident.

Chauncey turns out to be good at the French horn, and his music teacher is pleased. Yet he still wants to learn the trombone.

When he begins eighth grade, he tells his teacher he's not going to play French horn anymore, and he plans to take up the trombone. This leads to a discussion among Chauncey, his parents, and the music teacher. The teacher tells Chauncey and his parents what a talented French horn player he is, and he will leave a big hole in the school band if he switches instruments.

Chauncey is adamant, however, and his parents, to their credit, uphold their promise and support him.

Chauncey learns the new instrument quickly, and by the end of eighth grade, he has become the best trombonist in the band. However, the music teacher is angry that his parents stuck to their commitment to Chauncey and set aside the needs of the band. The music teacher holds a grudge and becomes passive-aggressive with Chauncey. He rarely praises Chauncey, criticizes him often, and offers him no help or instruction.

Chauncey knows he is a talented musician. Yet he has no interest in allowing himself to be so mistreated. At the end of the eighth grade, he quits the band, puts down the trombone, and never takes up another instrument.

## AMY AND HER MOTHER

Seven-year-old Amy goes to her mother for help in dealing with her hurting heart. Her friend Megan didn't invite her to her birthday party. However, six of her friends received invitations. Amy and Megan had always gone to each other's parties, so she is crushed and confused at not being invited.

Trish, Amy's mother, grew up during hard times. She learned to survive by being tough, practical, and thick-skinned. She wants to quickly soothe her daughter's pain and pass on some of her hard-earned wisdom and skills. So she tells her daughter, "Don't worry about it, honey. You have lots of friends! Besides, what Megan did says more about her than it does about you."

Trish thinks she is being helpful and teaching her daughter valuable survival skills.

However, that is not what Amy needs or is asking for right now. What she needs is to be listened to, believed, understood, cared for, and nurtured.

Her mom does none of these. Instead, Amy senses that her mother is dismissing her feelings and doesn't want her to be sad.

And young Amy is right. Trish is very uncomfortable with her daughter's sadness. She never learned how to deal with her own sadness, let alone Amy's.

When Amy doesn't get the nurturing she asks for, she feels rejected and not permitted to be who she is.

Trish tells her daughter, "You know what you can do, honey? Instead of worrying about Megan, you can think about something else, or go have fun with one of your other friends."

This is a classic EN move. Because Trish feels uncomfortable with Amy's pain, she encourages her daughter to distract herself from that pain so that Trish won't feel so uncomfortable.

However, Amy *already* feels that pain, and she wants that pain acknowledged and understood. Yet this is what Trish, caught in a moment of EN, refuses to do.

Right now, Amy doesn't think anyone understands her. She feels alone at school, forced out from her group of friends. Because of her mother's response, she now also feels alone at home, with a mother who doesn't seem to fully understand or care.

If this is an isolated incident, Amy will heal from it fairly quickly. However, if Trish continues to teach her to be tough and logical, and to not give her own feelings much credence, she will learn that it's not okay to be sad, to talk about her sadness, or to let herself get hurt. Amy will fear that she will be rejected once again if she does open up honestly about her feelings. Instead, she may learn to pretend that all is well inside her, even when it isn't. This will deeply embed EN in her heart.

Trish has put her own feelings ahead of her daughter's. As Amy grows older, if this becomes a pattern, she will learn that asking to be heard or discussing how she feels will lead quickly to her mother's disapproval. Eventually Amy may stop trying to talk about her feelings to anyone. She may never learn to take care of her feelings and her emotional life. Myths 1, 3, and 5 may reign within her heart.

## Myth 4: Following the Rules Is Also More Important than Addressing Our Needs and Feelings

Rules are necessary for any society to function. We see the value of rules when we drive in rush-hour traffic. Despite all the cars on the highway, rules enable us to get to our destinations without incident.

Contrast this with a big-box store such as Costco, where there are few rules for traffic flow—and where there are often bottlenecks or points of temporary chaos, as well as occasional cart collisions. When reasonable rules are followed, they create safety and predictability and make life easier.

Unfortunately, most of us never challenge the rules we learned as children. We simply accept and live by all of them, regardless of whether they help us or harm us. For example, we may automatically obey anyone in authority—a teacher, a spiritual leader, a coach, our boss—even after we have seen them abuse their authority.

Following rules—and demanding that others follow them— turns out to be one of the most painful, effective, and invisible ways in which we pass our EN to others, and they pass their EN to us. The two are so intertwined that I've devoted Chapter 5 to a detailed discussion of the topic.

## Myth 5: We Are Not Lovable as We Are; We Can Only Become Lovable through What We Do and Say

As we grow up according to the first four myths, and as everyday narcissism embeds itself ever deeper into our psyche, we eventually begin to intuit Myth 5. Through our parents' and other adults' EN, we learn at a young age that we are not inherently lovable just by being ourselves. Only if we do what adults want us to, follow their rules, and please them will we be considered lovable. Yet each time we are valued only for what we do and who we pretend to be, rather than for who we are, a wound is created or deepened.

Almost all of us figure out at a very young age that if we are obedient and compliant, then we're good and will be rewarded; if we're disobedient, we're bad and will be punished. Often the punishment for not being what others want is simple disapproval, or silence, or a sigh, or a look of judgment; sometimes, though, it takes the form of harsh words or violence. This is how adults, often unconsciously, control us and shape us into people who learn to take care of *their* needs and ignore our own.

## ADAM

By age ten, Adam has already faithfully internalized all the myths and principles of EN. He also diligently follows all the rules that adults expect him to follow. He has learned how to behave "perfectly" at all times. He follows directions and always says please and thank you. He is extremely responsible for a ten-year-old. Strangers who meet him praise him for acting like a little adult.

Adam's teachers love him because he is so easy to have in the classroom. Parents like to have Adam over because he adheres to all their rules and expectations, with no arguments.

Adam gets a lot of positive reinforcement for *not* being himself—for being a "good boy." In fact, however, Adam has learned to be a robot. He lives Myths 1, 3, 4, and 5 to perfection.

For the next two years, Adam's outward behavior doesn't change. One day, however, his father discovers a sketchbook hidden under his son's bed. In the sketchbook are many drawings of a boy sitting alone and looking very sad, holding a knife to his wrist, as if to cut himself. Inside the spiral binding of the sketchbook are three joints.

Adam's parents are shocked. They had no clue about their son's unhappiness. To them, he seemed like such a happy, well-adjusted boy. They wonder what has suddenly gone so wrong with their son. Adam's father blames the change on the early stirrings of adolescence.

In fact, something very right is beginning to happen inside Adam. He is starting to challenge the myths of EN and beginning to say to himself, "I'm *not* a robot. I do have feelings. I'm tired of existing just to make adults happy. I want desperately to matter. Somebody please acknowledge *me*."

Here is what makes Myth 5 especially toxic and insidious: the more we work to fulfill adults' needs, *the more we reinforce our own belief that we are not intrinsically lovable.* We learn to blame ourselves whenever we feel rejected. We tell ourselves that we must not be sufficiently smart, or lovable, or respectful, or obedient, or helpful; if we were, the people around us would feel happy and love us, rather than reject us.

> Human beings are wired to be connected in authentic ways, not false or trivial ones.

Since we've come to believe that we are not lovable as we are, we learn to hide our true self from other people. We create a public persona—a false self—who looks, speaks, and acts the way we think other people want us to. We develop a façade to ensure that we will be liked, accepted, and valued. Meanwhile, we live in fear that someone may find out what's behind that façade. We learn to live a lie.

This false self is then accepted by other false selves. Together, these false selves have created a world of partial, inauthentic connections. These connections are, understandably, less than satisfying. Human beings are wired to be connected in authentic ways, not false or trivial ones.

Because everyday narcissism is so widespread, here is the world it has helped us to create:

- We spend our days trying desperately to belong. We focus on doing and being what everyone else wants us to do or be—or, at least, what we *think* they want us to do or be.

- This focus requires us to discount ourselves and deny our own truth—day by day, moment after moment, over and over. This takes away much of our freedom and energy. It deprives us of the joy of exploring, searching, challenging, adventuring, and discovering ourselves. It undermines our self-esteem and self-confidence.

- We yearn for genuine connections with other people, yet we may not know how to create such connections. We only know how to create inauthentic ones, by reaching out from one false self to another.

- Or, perhaps, we *do* know how to create these connections—yet we don't dare attempt them. We're terrified that if we do show people our real self, they will reject us and turn away in disgust. We fear that we will then lose what little, limited, inauthentic connection we had with them.

- Or, maybe we've never been fortunate enough to have *ever* experienced an authentic connection with another human being. We may not know what such a connection looks or feels like. We may not even realize that such a relationship is possible.

- Or, we may think the paltry connections that false selves have with one another *are* intimacy, and they are the best we can offer one another.

- Yet, at the same time, something inside us tells us that all of this isn't enough. Although we may not be able to put words to the feeling, we yearn for something more, something real, something authentic.

- We are exhausted from our attempts to maintain the lies we live by.

## The Need to Belong

These five myths create innumerable childhood wounds. When we repeatedly experience our needs as unimportant, we eventually come to believe that *we* are unimportant.

When kids attempt to fulfill their own needs, and those attempts conflict with an adult's desires—or, often, a rule—the adult typically responds with judgment, anger, an expression of dismay ("I'm so disappointed in you"), and rejection. Over time, children thus learn to ignore, deny, or discount their own needs. They also learn to believe Myths 3 and 4.

We all have a basic need to belong, to not be rejected by others—especially by our parents and other powerful adults in our life. As a result, to avoid rejection, many of us learned at an early age to focus our efforts on pleasing other people. However, some of us did the opposite. When our efforts to get approval failed, we became defiant, hoping to salvage a bit of self-esteem. Still others tried to become invisible as a way to avoid others' judgment and rejection.

Whatever our childhood survival pattern was, it all came from the same need to be loved, to count, and to matter—that is, to belong. Myths 3 and 4 teach us the opposite: that we don't matter very much. They also teach us that, in order to matter to adults, we need to subordinate ourselves to their desires and rules.

> Whatever our childhood survival pattern was,
> it all came from the same need to be loved, to
> count, and to matter—that is, to belong.

As we grow up, we internalize and normalize these messages. We take them for granted, believe they are true and inevitable, and assume nothing can be done to change them. We get so used to being verbally abused that we tell ourselves it is no big deal, just a part of life. We normalize not being seen as important, not being heard, not having our needs met. As a result, we become more and more angry, more and more depressed, and more and more anxious.

Eventually, as we learn to live our lives according to these myths, we don't take time for ourselves. We get so focused on others that we lose our ability to even know what we want, what will make us happy, or what would be fun. We stop having dreams of our own. Some of us become martyrs.

Meanwhile, we regularly pass on these same messages to others—including our own children.

## Our Myth-Centered Worldview

Up until now, I've written about how the five myths affect our interactions with each other. However, their effects go well beyond person-to-person relationships. They also warp how we view our place in the universe. As they become embedded in our minds and hearts, they create a worldview based on the following assumptions:

- The world—laws, social and religious norms, commerce, communication, even the weather—is supposed to revolve around me.

- It's the job of life (or God, or the universe) to make me happy. I'm entitled to happiness.

- When I'm not happy or things don't go well for me, I'm entitled to feel betrayed by life and act like an angry victim.

These assumptions are largely unconscious. Most of us have no idea they are running—and sometimes ruining—our lives. Yet none of them is remotely true. And it's easy to recognize the narcissism embedded in them.

Just as we can't make other human beings do and say and be what we want, we can't coax the world into compliance with our desires. We can do good deeds; we can pray; we can follow all the rules; and we can do our best. Yet, whatever we do, sometimes we get the results we want, and sometimes we don't. Or, as Rabbi Rami Shapiro puts it, our prayers are always answered—and sometimes the answer is *no*.

> . . . we can't coax the world into compliance
> with our desires.

The world does not exist to make us happy. Life is often hard, painful, or disappointing—and sometimes all three.

This is not a new or radical insight. It is sometimes called *the tragic vision*, which has been widely noted and discussed by writers, theologians, and philosophers for centuries. (In recent decades, M. Scott Peck and Thomas Sowell have both written eloquently on the subject.) It is also one of the foundational principles of psychotherapy.

I've traveled all around the world. When I visited Jordan, Bhutan, Russia, and other countries that don't have the wealth, opportunity, political freedoms, or relatively mild weather that we have in most of the United States, here's what struck me: *people in those countries completely accept that life is hard*. They don't question this reality, or ask or expect or demand that life be otherwise.

Although life is usually less harrowing in rich and relatively safe nations, it is *still* difficult and painful—because that is the nature of life. Yet we often do our best to shy away from this basic reality.

The unrealistic view that the job of the world (and/or God) is to make us happy results in our feeling miserable and like a victim— and it is yet another compelling reason to heal from our EN.

Sometimes in my therapy office, a client will say to me, "Nancy, I'm angry with God. My life just isn't what I want it to be."

I usually nod and say, "It sounds to me like God's been talking to you, and you've not liked what you've heard, so you've been ignoring the wisdom you've been given. Perhaps that has created part of the problem. Maybe it's time to try listening and trusting."

## The Promise

Fortunately, there's an alternative to a life built around everyday narcissism. Each of us can heal from our EN and the problems it creates. We can recover from our childhood wounds and from the habits and patterns we developed to fit in and survive.

We can discover a path back to who we truly are. We can find an authentic way to live—a way in which we belong, and are loved, and are seen as worthy for who we truly are.

I promise you that so much more is possible.

## Our Need to Belong

Our need to belong is one of the most powerful of human drives.

More than a century ago, Sigmund Freud posited that our strongest drive was sex. His protégé Alfred Adler, who broke away from Freud in 1918, disagreed. He believed that our greatest drive was our need to belong, to be loved, to be liked, to be a part of a community.

In 1943, psychologist Abraham Maslow proposed a *hierarchy of needs*. According to Maslow, human beings' most basic needs are food, shelter, and clothing. Just above that is safety—and immediately above that is the need to belong and to be loved.

Our desire to belong is so strong that we will do almost anything to fulfill it. We will live by painful, life-denying myths and principles. We will give up many of our values and forms of meaning. We will sacrifice our freedom. We will do without the joy of self-exploration, searching, challenging, discovering, and having adventures. We will let our wings be clipped. We will deny who we are and pretend to be who we are not, all just to belong.

## Creating Emotional Safety

As we've seen, everyday narcissism creates an endless and fruitless quest to be accepted and cared for by others. It causes us to believe that we are not inherently lovable or valuable, and that we don't really belong—and, perhaps, that we don't *deserve* to belong.

In addition, because of our own EN, and the EN of others around us, we don't feel emotionally safe. Being our authentic self feels risky and dangerous. After all, when we were younger and didn't know how to be anyone other than our true self, we were repeatedly judged and rejected. We were told to change, to be different, to be what others wanted us to be—because who we really were was inadequate and unworthy of love.

Over time, we create a false self in the hope of becoming safe and loved. We became what others wanted (or what we believed others wanted) us to be—a pleaser, a peacemaker, a good girl or boy—all in an attempt to belong and feel safe. Yet we never do actually manage to feel safe, because we carry inside us the inevitable fear of being found out—of others discovering that we're a phony. Then, we fear, we will *definitely* be rejected for good.

Meanwhile, we try to feel safer by making inauthentic connections between our own false self and the false selves of others. Yet each such connection only leaves us feeling even *more* unsafe, because a part of us remains acutely aware of the lies and myths on which such connections are built.

Eventually the world, its inhabitants, and its situations all seem inherently frightening and dangerous. We live in more-or-less constant fear of others' rejection and judgment. As a result, some of us struggle with depression or anxiety. Almost all of us become somewhat neurotic.

*Neuroses* are a class of mechanisms people develop to cope with stress. These mechanisms are dysfunctional, yet they usually fall within socially acceptable limits.

Typical neuroses include shyness, extreme quietness, perfectionism, anxiousness, and, of course, compulsively pleasing others. One common neurosis involves always attempting to get things *right*: to have the right car, clothes, job, friends, and hairstyle; to live in the right neighborhood; to go to the right college; to work in the right job or career; and so on. Other common neuroses involve being arrogant, aggressive, bossy, or bullying.

All of these are common, "normal" accommodations to the fears and myths we carry inside us. They are usually our unconscious attempt to create the emotional safety we so desperately crave. And these accommodations *can* sometimes protect us, temporarily and provisionally, from the judgment of others. However, no accommodation can give us a lasting sense of emotional safety. *Genuine safety can only come from being our authentic self.* Only by living out of that self—and being vulnerable to the slings and arrows of others—is real safety possible.

Paradoxically, *actual* emotional safety involves not requiring others to accept, respect, like, or love us. Instead, it requires that we accept, respect, like, and love *ourselves*—and trust our own ability to take care of ourselves emotionally.

> Genuine safety can only come from being
> our authentic self.

Emotional safety is not something we need to beg, wheedle, or otherwise acquire from others. Instead, we must learn to create it for ourselves. We do this by being our authentic self and learning to trust the wisdom, desires, and inclinations of that self.

## Making the Turn

Each of us can heal from our EN and the problems it creates. This healing is the subject of the remainder of this book.

Your healing begins with challenging the myths that have been integral parts of your life for so many years. It means facing your fear of rejection and learning to speak your truth with kindness, honesty, and graciousness. It means being true to yourself and giving up the pretenses and expectations others placed on you. In this process, you will lose some relationships because, suddenly, you will stop focusing on pleasing other people.

> Your healing begins with challenging the myths that have been integral parts of your life for so many years.

For a time, this will make you somewhat unpredictable to others, some of whom will initially feel less safe around you. Others, however, will grow to trust and respect you more because they will feel they can count on your honesty and authenticity.

The people who genuinely care about you will stick around and will appreciate your efforts to grow and heal. They will love you for who you are instead of who you may have pretended to be.

As part of this process of healing and growth, you will investigate your own EN and the myths you have been taught. You will also learn to stop writing mental stories about what you think other people are going to do or feel in response to what you do. And you will begin to forgive yourself and bring compassion to the wounds you carry.

More important still, you will learn to live in the moment. You will stop trying to control everything (because you can't; no one can). And you will let go of the outcomes of your choices.

This can be scary at first. However, it is an important part of creating an authentic life. You will also begin to live into these truths:

- You are not responsible for how others feel or act; you *are*, however, responsible for how *you* feel and act.
- You are also responsible for living in your truth—with kindness and graciousness.

- Others are not responsible for your happiness and serenity; *you* are.

- *You* are important. You do count. You are inherently lovable as you are.

- You do not need to try to be what others want you to be.

- Like everyone else, you have things to learn about life and what will make it rich for you.

Let the healing begin.

---

## HEALING ACTIVITY #1

---

### Become Aware of the Five Myths

Cut out or copy the list of the five myths at the beginning of this book. Post this list in a spot where you can see it regularly: on a home bulletin board, on the outside of a kitchen cupboard, near your desk at work, or on the dashboard of your car.

If you like, also cut out or copy the card-sized list of myths at the end of this book and carry it with you in your wallet or purse.

Review the list at least once or twice each day, until you can easily recall all five myths.

---

## HEALING ACTIVITY #2

---

### Notice the Five Myths as You Go About Your Day

As you go through your day, notice whenever someone uses one or more of the following words or phrases. These are all expressions of one or more of the myths of EN.

- You made me screw up/late/trip and fall/etc.

- You make me angry/upset/nervous/infuriated/etc.

- You ruined my day/the party/our anniversary/etc.

- I wouldn't have gotten so angry/yelled/thrown the chair/etc. if you hadn't . . .

- I'll feel better/happier/more comfortable/less uncomfortable if you do what I say/do what I want/ keep quiet/etc.

- I'm so disappointed you didn't . . .

- Don't feel that way.

- You're too emotional/sensitive/thin-skinned/etc.

- It's wrong/stupid/foolish/childish to feel or think that way.

When you recognize that one of these myths is being expressed, say to yourself, *That's not true. That's a myth.* Also see if you can identify the particular myth or myths. Often it will be more than one.

Do this until noticing the myths of EN becomes second nature.

## HEALING ACTIVITY #3

### Notice When You Fall into the Five Myths of EN

Once you have begun to notice when others are acting out of EN, the next step is to become aware of EN in your own thoughts, speech, and actions. You can't change what you do until you become aware of what you're doing. This healing activity can help you become more aware of yourself.

Listen to yourself as you talk to others. Each time you hear one of the myths coming out of your own mouth, congratulate yourself for catching it. Then stop and say to whomever you're talking to, "Wait a second. That's not what I wanted to say. Let me try again."

Then mentally replay what you said. If it sounds like one of the statements from Healing Activity #2, restate what you want or believe in way that is respectful of yourself *and* the other person. Here are some examples.

| INSTEAD OF | YOU MIGHT SAY |
|---|---|
| Now I'm late because of you. That's really going to mess up my afternoon. | I chose to keep talking to you, so now I'm late. Got to go. Catch you later! |
| You made me really happy with this gift. | I'm very happy with this gift. |
| I'm so disappointed that you didn't do your math homework. | I'm concerned you didn't do your math homework because math is an important skill you'll need in order to do well in life. |
| Give Grandma a kiss goodbye. | Would you like to give Grandma a kiss goodbye? |
| Thank Jane for the delicious dinner, even if you didn't like it. It's the polite thing to do. | Would you like to thank Jane for fixing us dinner and having us over? |
| Just stand quietly next to me, hold my arm, and smile. That's what everyone wants and expects. | The world expects you to be my arm candy. I just want you to be yourself. |

Once you've learned to regularly notice when the myths of EN show up in what you say, you'll be equipped to start noticing when you write them in texts, emails, and other messages. As soon as you recognize such a message, catch yourself, congratulate yourself on your awareness and insight, and rewrite what you've written so that it respects both you and your recipient.

The next step is to watch for and notice when the myths appear in the things you *think*. When you notice you've fallen into EN thinking, catch and correct your thoughts in the same way you learned to do with your spoken and written words.

All of these powerful practices can spare you and others a great deal of misery.

# 4

# Building Boundaries

"Let your heart guide you.
It whispers, so listen closely."

*The Land Before Time*

Who we are is made up of our likes, dislikes, wants, needs, feelings, values, beliefs, experiences, and spirituality. These comprise our personal boundaries—our truths. The myths of EN tell us these truths are not important. Instead, we are encouraged to live by others' truths because those are supposedly more important than our own.

As we grow up and begin to live according to the myths of EN, we lose sight of who we are. Instead, we focus on taking care of others and being responsible for them. When we do this, we become boundaryless. We conform ourselves to what others ask and expect of us. We change who we appear to be, much like a chameleon, to fit in and be accepted.

When we don't express who we truly are through our actions or words, we fail to declare ourselves. We don't express our boundaries, our identity, our truth—either to others or to ourselves. When we eat food we dislike, have sex when we don't want to, or outwardly agree to something we don't inwardly agree with, we have violated our own boundary. We have not honored ourselves.

Some of us partly honor ourselves and then stop and freeze. We say what we want and what is important to us; however, we don't actually do anything about it. We may complain about not getting what we want or need, yet we don't seriously attempt to fulfill that need or desire on our own. We wait for the other person to change, to give us what we want. We don't take the risk of acting or changing ourselves.

> Each time we don't honor our own boundaries,
> and each time others don't honor who we are,
> an old wound is deepened.

Over time, when we repeatedly fail to fully honor ourselves, many of us no longer know who we are. We only know what others want us to be. We become so focused on others' desires that we don't know our own truth or trust the wisdom in it or live by our own values. And, of course, we don't set our own boundaries. Yet, at the same time, a part of us remains innately in touch with our own truth. This innate wisdom leads to anger when we are not respected, either by others or ourselves.

Each time we don't honor our own boundaries, and each time others don't honor who we are, an old wound is deepened. As a result, anger and hurt get stored inside us. As children, many of us keep this anger and hurt to ourselves. To our young minds, expressing those feelings would result in rejection. And, often, we'd be right. We do this over and over until we come to believe we don't even have a right to feel angry or hurt.

## RUTH AND HAL

By the time Ruth turns fifteen, she has learned from her parents, her grandparents, her teachers, and most other adults that she has the power and the responsibility to make everyone else happy.

Ruth is in ninth grade. Her parents and teachers are proud of her. She studies hard, earns high grades, and is active in her synagogue. She is not particularly interested in school or Judaism; however, she knows how to please the adults in her life. What Ruth loves to do for herself is draw and paint, and she is grateful that her relatives and teachers consider this an acceptable activity.

One day Hal, a boy from the neighborhood, asks her out to a movie. She doesn't know him very well. Her parents and his parents are friends, though, so she says yes.

Ruth enjoys the movie; however, she finds Hal selfish and boring. As he drives her home after the film, he talks about himself in great detail and does not ask her any questions about herself or her life.

After Hal parks the car near her home, he tries to kiss her. She says, "No, Hal," and turns her head away. He says, "Oh, come on," takes her head in his hands, and plants a firm kiss on her mouth.

She pushes him away. "Hey! I said no." She attempts to set a clear, firm boundary.

Not respecting that boundary, Hal leans toward her and says, "Don't be so cold to me. I like you. You don't want to hurt my feelings, do you?"

This confuses Ruth. She believes she has a right to say no. Suddenly, though, all the EN myths come flooding into her mind. She wants to be liked and accepted—by Hal, by his parents, and by people in general. She's afraid that Hal won't like her if she keeps holding him off, even if she doesn't like him that much. In her fear, she disregards her own boundaries. So she gives in to his kisses, and she and Hal make out in the car for several minutes.

> Later, alone in her bedroom, Ruth feels sad, confused, bewildered, and disappointed in herself. She doesn't understand why she spent five minutes kissing a boy she doesn't like.

## EN and Chronic Passivity

One common variant of failing to honor our own boundaries is passivity. There are times in everyone's life when passiveness—being patient, waiting and seeing, taking a step back, or letting someone else take the lead—can be wise. For some of us, though, EN encourages us to make passiveness a way of life. We let others set our goals, guide us, and tell us what to do. We rarely or never state what we want or need. We don't take responsibility for ourselves or our feelings.

Passivity is like being a leaf in the river; it just flows with the current. That current may take the leaf down the rapids, or slam up it against a log, or wash it up on a random beach. Whatever happens, though, we get to tell ourselves that we weren't to blame, that what happened was done *to* us. That's the emotional payoffs of passivity.

Conflict avoidance is perhaps the most common form of passivity. For many of us, conflict is frightening. As children, conflict may have usually resulted in feeling rejected, hurt, and alone—so we learned to avoid it as much as we could, often by keeping quiet.

Yet conflict is an unavoidable part of life. When we try to avoid conflict, we create a new conflict within ourselves. As a result, tension forms around that conflict. This tension is not between us and another person; it's inside us. Then we become upset or angry about what may or may not happen. Because we keep this conflict inside ourselves, there's no risk of rejection. That's the payoff for us. Yet if we regularly repeat this behavior—and, if we're conflict avoidant, we probably will—then, over time, our anger collects, and our resentments build. This often leads to depression.

Furthermore, when we repeatedly avoid conflict, we tend to let others take advantage of us. This only adds to our anger and resentment.

Eventually something inside us rebels. It can no longer tolerate not being counted, not being listened to. We may suddenly blow our top and lash out. Either we lash out at others or we get angry with ourselves for not speaking up. Then we punish ourselves, become depressed, or both.

In short, when we choose conflict avoidance, we might manage to avoid immediate discomfort. However, we usually create long-term misery.

When adults are chronically conflict avoidant, that form of passivity often began as a sensible adaptation to a childhood in which most conflicts led to them being harmed or rejected. They learned they were better off giving in than standing up for themselves.

Paradoxically, some chronically avoidant adults were feisty children who *did* regularly stand up for themselves. However, their parents repeatedly punished or rejected them for their feistiness—and they eventually surrendered.

Other chronically avoidant adults were born with more passive natures. Many of these people struggled with asserting themselves from a very young age. Now they rarely stand up for what they want or need, and they tend to cave in easily, get discouraged easily, and have little resilience. They have learned to take whatever life offers, the good and the bad, and don't usually ask for—or work for—anything different.

When faced with conflict as adults, chronically passive people tend to get better and better at becoming silent and not making waves. Whether this passivity is partly natural or 100 percent learned, two common EN fears are behind it: a fear of becoming vulnerable and a fear of being rejected if they speak their truth, or take a stand that might displease someone.

Often there is another EN lesson behind passivity: if we believe that other people are ultimately responsible for our happiness, then there is no need to advocate for ourselves. We get to be irresponsible about creating our own happiness—and we get to blame others when we're feeling down or when things don't go our way.

Yet chronic passivity is never an adequate response to life. There are times when each of us needs to get a canoe and a paddle, put them into the river, and start paddling and steering in the direction we want our life to go.

Passive people do get angry, of course. However, they usually don't express much of their anger outwardly; they just feel it silently and express it indirectly, through pouting, sideways comments, ignoring others, refusing to speak to people, simply going away or leaving relationships, and so on.

## LINDSAY AND FELIPE

Lindsay came to therapy very distressed and sad. Her marriage of forty years had just ended.

In May her husband made her a beautiful Mother's Day card, in which he expounded on his love for her. Three weeks later he told her he was seeking a divorce.

Lindsay was understandably in shock. She told me she and her husband never fought, and she was always able to say clearly what she wanted in the marriage. In fact, she felt that in many ways their marriage was ideal. Yet clearly it had been otherwise.

Eventually, through my sessions with Lindsay, I discovered that her husband, Felipe, was chronically passive. He almost never stood up for what he wanted and usually deferred to her wishes. What Lindsay saw as similar interests and great compatibility was Felipe's passive agreement to whatever she wanted. After four decades of not getting his needs met, because he rarely made them known, Felipe was bursting with anger and resentment. He blamed Lindsay for most of his unhappiness, so he decided to leave, imagining that once she was out of his life, happiness would magically appear.

Even in filing for divorce, Felipe was still being passive. Instead of telling Lindsay what he needed and wanted, or even being willing to talk about what had been bothering him, he simply announced that the marriage was over and left.

## Crisis Points

As we live according to the myths and principles of EN, and as we continue to dishonor ourselves and permit others to dishonor us, our unexpressed anger builds. With each boundary violation we experience, we add another stone of anger to the pile.

One day the anger becomes too much. Something—often some very small emotional wounding—occurs, and suddenly we are triggered. One of three things typically occurs:

- We explode, spontaneously expressing years of unexpressed anger. Suddenly we are telling someone about all the things they've said or done that hurt or angered us. We blame them for our misery and, perhaps, accuse them of being a terrible human being. Meanwhile, we don't take responsibility for own decision to not stay true to ourselves. This explosion feels good because the internal pressure has been released. Soon afterward, though, we may realize we were unkind, unfair, or even cruel in how we expressed our anger. Remorse may then set in. In this scenario, we walk away still wounded, now having wounded someone else as well. Meanwhile, nothing has been resolved.

- We implode, getting deeply angry with ourselves for not speaking up and allowing ourselves to be mistreated. Then we become seriously depressed.

- We explode *and* implode. We blame the other person for our misery *and* we get angry with ourselves for letting others treat us so poorly, for not speaking our truth, or for not standing up for ourselves.

## Honoring Your Truth

Now, however, you have an opportunity to break this cycle. You can learn to honor your truth and openly express yourself to others—without either exploding or imploding. You can learn how to express yourself to others with a combination of honesty, kindness, and graciousness. This means

- challenging the lies inherent in the myths and principles of EN;

- taking full responsibility for your own happiness;

- being willing to walk into conflict;

- accepting your fear and moving forward in the face of it (this is the very definition of courage);

- learning to say difficult things to people in a respectful and loving way;

- being assertive without being aggressive or accusatory;

- no longer pointing your finger at others and telling them what you feel *they* need to do or say;

- focusing and acting on what *you* need, want, and feel;

- letting go of blame;

- listening to your heart, and your truth, again and again—and living in that truth;

- understanding that change takes time and involves some mistakes and setbacks;

- focusing on progress, not perfection.

Change is uncomfortable, often scary, and sometimes terrifying. At first, you'll fear that the changes you're going through will limit your ability to belong, to fit in, to be a part of some group or community. In fact, they will do exactly the opposite—though you may eventually find yourself belonging to a different group.

> . . . it is important to pay attention to your body and let yourself make mistakes, apologizing when appropriate.

As you read the rest of this book and move through this process, you won't know what the outcome will look like. You will enter entirely new territory. This is wonderful because it offers an alternative to living according to the EN myths that have created so much unhappiness in your life.

Throughout this process of learning, changing, and growing, it is important to pay attention to your body and let yourself make mistakes, apologizing when appropriate.

# HEALING ACTIVITY #4

## Pay Attention to Your Body

The human body is a very wise organism. It is designed to survive and has done so for many thousands of years. Your own body will send you signals all the time; pay attention to them. For example, when someone asks you to do something, your body will let you know if it is right for you to do it.

If fear arises, pay attention to it *briefly*—for only thirty seconds or less. View it as a warning. Listen to the wisdom of that warning and take action accordingly. However, never let fear alone make a decision for you. Often our fear comes from the scared little person inside us who fears rejection.

If you're unsure of what your body is telling you, stop what you're doing for a moment. If necessary, say to the person or people you are with, "Give me just a moment, please." If necessary, turn away or leave the room. Then simply stand or sit quietly. Cast your gaze downward and take two or three deep, slow breaths. This will help you access what your body is telling you. Listen.

You will need time and practice to learn to listen to what your body tells you in order to access its wisdom. Internally test out each possible response; over time, you'll be able to feel which one is right for you.

Please pay particular attention to anger and fear. These emotions can quickly close our hearts, and when our hearts are closed, we cannot connect to ourselves, let alone to others. Yet when we don't cling to or feed anger and fear, they can subside as quickly as they arise.

When we get angry with our children and say harsh things to them, our hearts are closed, and we are disconnected from both their hearts and our own. Yet ten minutes later, once our anger has subsided, our heart starts to open again.

We reconnect to our heart, feel love for our kids once again, and feel badly for what we said or did.

---

## HEALING ACTIVITY #5

---

## Let Yourself Make Mistakes—
## And Apologize When Appropriate

As you honor and speak your truth, you will rediscover who you are, which people in your life genuinely care about you, and which ones do not. The ones who care will understand when you make a mistake and will normally accept a genuine apology.

It's important to speak your truth—and to do so graciously. You probably wouldn't say to your best friend, "That outfit looks awful on you"; instead, you'd more likely say, "I don't think that's as flattering as some of your other outfits. If you like it, though, that's what matters."

As you practice speaking your truth, sometimes you may unwittingly do so in an unkind way. This doesn't mean it was wrong to express yourself honestly—only that it's important to practice kindness and compassion at the same time.

For example, if you shout at your friend, "Back off, damn it! Stop badgering me!" you honored yourself by setting a boundary. However, you also dishonored your friend—and yourself—by shouting and swearing. Instead, you might have said softly, "I've heard what you want. Thanks for telling me. Now I need to stop talking about this."

When you do speak unkindly, I recommend a simple and honest apology. However, don't apologize for speaking your truth, or getting angry, or being who you are. None of these requires an apology. Instead, say something like, "I'm not sorry I got angry. I'm sorry for the way I expressed my anger, though. That must have hurt."

## What You Need to Know About Your Emotions

Behind all the myths and principles of EN is this unrealistic expectation: *don't have your own emotions or needs, because they make other people uncomfortable.*

When we are young, the most significant "other people" in our lives are our parents. Very likely they were not allowed to have their own emotions and needs as children, either. As a result, they didn't know how to take care of their own feelings. And so, EN gets passed down from generation to generation, like a genetically inherited illness. In addition, because we don't have much access to our emotions or know much about how to take care of them, we generally have ineffective boundaries.

Because of EN, most of us were never taught how to take care of our own hearts—or how to know and communicate our own emotional needs. When we experience sensations in our body, we don't know how to understand what they tell us. Instead, we may have learned to disconnect from our own body—and, therefore, our emotions.

> Our emotions hold—or embody—a great deal
> of wisdom. We need to learn to listen to them.

Emotions are not ideas. They are intensely physical, the language of the body. Our emotions hold—or embody—a great deal of wisdom. We need to learn to listen to them.

Letting ourselves fully experience our emotions is a huge step toward healing and happiness. It also helps prepares our heart to forgive. Part of experiencing these emotions is naming them.

---

## HEALING ACTIVITY #6

---

### Listen To and Name Your Feelings

A helpful and empowering first step is clearly recognizing and acknowledging each emotion. Because, over the years, you've learned to ignore your heart and your emotions, it may be difficult at first for you to recognize and name them, beyond *hurt*, *sad*, *happy*, and *mad*.

Deliberately naming your feelings may feel strange, awkward, uncomfortable, or difficult. However, with time and practice it will become easier and faster—until, one day, it becomes nearly effortless and instantaneous. In the process, you will discover a lot of valuable information about yourself. Your emotional vocabulary will increase dramatically, and your ability to care for yourself and communicate with others will increase tenfold.

When you can name each emotion, you can then choose how to best deal with it. This makes you more able to take care of yourself. For example, if you know you feel lonely, you can call a friend, join a club or group, or do something else to feel less lonely. If you are feeling unsafe, you can take steps to feel safer. As you listen to how you feel and what your heart is telling you, your heart will start to open. Your body will start to trust you and your ability to care for it.

To help you build this skill, please do the following brief activity at least once a day. If possible, do it in the afternoon or evening, so you can reflect back on most of the day's events.

- Find a notebook that feels good to you. This can be a bound, blank book; a binder; a diary; or any other well-made, physical book. You will be putting your heart into this book, so make sure it can handle plenty of use and its pages will not fall out over time. Also, the book should be something you like looking at, that feels good in your hands, and that you can easily write in and carry with you. This will become your healing notebook.

- If you like, put the myths and false principles of EN on the cover or the first page, for easy reference.

- Find a place where you can sit by yourself, quietly and comfortably. Bring with you this book; a pencil, pen, or marker; and your healing notebook.

- Turn to the back of this book, where you'll find a list of feelings. Read this entire list from beginning to end. (No skimming or short cuts, please.)

- Cast your gaze downward and sit quietly, simply breathing and feeling into your body, for three to five minutes. (Looking down is important. When you look up, you will access information in your brain, not your heart.)

- Write today's date at the top of a new page in your healing notebook.

- Mentally review your day from when you woke until this moment and write down all the feelings you experienced so far.

- Quickly review the feelings list again. If you see another emotion you experienced during the day that is not yet in that day's notebook entry, write it down now.

- Write down as many feelings as you can name—at least six, and preferably more. (If you have trouble coming up with six, review the feelings list again and sit quietly for a few more minutes. Be patient with yourself and allow the emotions to emerge.)

- Be as complete as you can. The more feelings you list, the more details you are giving yourself about your life and your inner experience.

- You may notice that multiple, or even opposing, feelings can arise at the same time. For example, you might feel both fear and anticipation, or happiness and disappointment. This is normal—and, in fact, quite common.

Write down your feelings in your healing notebook once a day until the practice becomes a familiar habit.

After that, continue to write down your feelings daily. In addition, check in with your heart and body every few hours, simply noting (without writing anything down) what you feel.

When you name your feelings each day in your notebook, you challenge the myths of EN. You announce to yourself that you do matter and that there are times when your own needs come first.

This can feel scary or overwhelming at first. That's okay. Let yourself feel scared or overwhelmed for a short time. Then take a few deep breaths and return to these healing activities.

---

## HEALING ACTIVITY #7

---

### Notice and Investigate Your Anger

Some people who grew up steeped in EN have trouble expressing their anger honestly and respectfully. If you struggle with expressing your anger, then, at least once a day, review the list of feelings and the list of angry feelings on the pages that follow (and that also appear at the back of this book). Include in your healing notebook all the emotions on this list that you experienced that day. *If you don't have difficulty expressing your anger, skip this activity.*

Remember that anger often hides or masks other underlying emotions. We frequently get angry after (or because) we feel embarrassed, or demeaned, or discounted, or betrayed. You'll discover it's enormously helpful to courageously embrace and fully feel these underlying emotions, such as embarrassment, humiliation, and betrayal. Doing this will help you know yourself better and take better care of yourself.

Staying in anger without looking at what may be underneath can prevent you from stepping into those underlying feelings, experiencing them fully in your body, and knowing yourself. Staying in the anger can be like seeing a physician for a persistent cough and asking for a cough suppressant, yet not allowing the doctor to check for the cough's underlying cause. If you have pneumonia, treating only the symptoms will make you sicker, not healthier. Similarly, feelings that go unaddressed can create serious problems such as depression, anxiety, aggressiveness, and a variety of physical ailments.

When you get angry, go ahead and feel that anger in your body for ten to fifteen seconds. This anger is useful: it tells you that something is wrong. If you stay in the anger too long, you can easily slide into Myth 2 and victim energy. Instead of remaining in the anger, be curious about it. Ask yourself what it is about, and look at any other feelings that may be behind or beneath it.

## FEELINGS

| | | |
|---|---|---|
| Abandoned | Blessed | Constricted |
| Affectionate | Blue | Content |
| Affirmed | Bored | Controlled |
| Afraid | Bound | Crappy |
| Alarmed | Brave | Crazy |
| Alive | Burdened | Crushed |
| Alone | Buzzed | Curious |
| Ambivalent | Calm | Deceived |
| Angry | Capable | Defeated |
| Anxious | Cared for | Defensive |
| Appalled | Carefree | Delighted |
| Appreciated | Certain | Demeaned |
| Appreciative | Charmed | Depressed |
| Apprehensive | Cheated | Despairing |
| Aroused | Cheerful | Desperate |
| Ashamed | Compassionate | Devastated |
| Bad | Concerned | Diminished |
| Bashful | Confident | Disappointed |
| Betrayed | Conflicted | Discounted |
| Bewildered | Confused | Discouraged |

| | | |
|---|---|---|
| Disempowered | Fearless | Ignored |
| Disgruntled | Firm | Impatient |
| Disgusted | Flushed | Imposed upon |
| Dismissive | Flustered | Impotent |
| Dissed | Fortunate | Inadequate |
| Distant | Frantic | Incapable |
| Distraught | Frenetic | Inept |
| Distressed | Frightened | Inferior |
| Distrustful | Gay | Inspired |
| Disturbed | Generous | Intimidated |
| Dominated | Giddy | Invisible |
| Doubtful | Glad | Isolated |
| Dumb | Grateful | Jealous |
| Eager | Grief-stricken | Joyful |
| Elated | Guilty | Jubilant |
| Embarrassed | Happy | Jumpy |
| Emboldened | Healthy | Kind |
| Empathetic | Held back | Left out |
| Empowered | Helpful | Listless |
| Empty | Helpless | Lonely |
| Encouraged | Hesitant | Lost |
| Energetic | High | Loved |
| Energized | Honored | Loving |
| Enervated | Hopeful | Melancholy |
| Entitled | Hopeless | Miserable |
| Envious | Humble | Motivated |
| Excited | Humiliated | Mournful |
| Exhausted | Hungry | Nauseated |
| Fearful | Hurt | Needed |

| | | |
|---|---|---|
| Needy | Scared | Trapped |
| Nervous | Self-righteous | Troubled |
| Numb | Sexy | Trusting |
| Open | Shaky | Uncertain |
| Oppressed | Shameful | Uneasy |
| Panicky | Shocked | Unappreciated |
| Patient | Shy | Unimportant |
| Passionate | Sick | Unloved |
| Peaceful | Sluggish | Unmotivated |
| Pleased | Somber | Unsafe |
| Powerful | Sorrowful | Unsure |
| Powerless | Stifled | Unworthy |
| Pressured | Stressed | Upset |
| Proud | Strong | Uptight |
| Put upon | Stuck | Used |
| Rejected | Stunned | Violated |
| Relaxed | Stupid | Vulnerable |
| Released | Suffocated | Wanted |
| Relieved | Supported | Weak |
| Remorseful | Sympathetic | Weary |
| Rested | Tense | Weepy |
| Restless | Terrified | Wimpy |
| Reticent | Thankful | Worn out |
| Revolted | Thrilled | Worried |
| Romantic | Thwarted | Worthy |
| Run down | Tickled | Wound up |
| Sad | Tight | Wrung out |
| Safe | Tired | |
| Satisfied | Tough | |

## ANGRY FEELINGS

| | | |
|---|---|---|
| Angry | Furious | Outraged |
| Annoyed | Hateful | Rageful |
| Cantankerous | Incensed | Resentful |
| Crabby | Indignant | Spiteful |
| Enraged | Infuriated | Ticked off |
| Exasperated | Irritated | Vengeful |
| Frustrated | Mad | |

## How EN Encourages Resentment

As we've seen, everyday narcissism teaches us to focus on what other people want us to do and be—and to ignore our own desires. So, as we grow up, many of us become proficient at pleasing others and recognizing what others want of us. We become pleasers. People really like us for this. Eventually pleasing others becomes a way of life and an identity.

Meanwhile, we ignore our own needs and desires. We also avoid conflict. We fear that any conflict with others will cause them to stop being pleased with us, and perhaps not like us. This is particularly true for women.

We also assume that doing all this will keep us safe and happy because we believe in Myth 2—that others will give us what we want and need in return. Of course, this doesn't work. And, over time, as others fail to live up to our expectations, we become angry and resentful.

---

### ROSA AND JOSÉ

Rosa came to her first appointment with me feeling confused, scared, furious, and depressed. For the past ten years, she had been taking antidepressants. She was not happy in her marriage and was considering having an affair. (That is never a good sign.)

Rosa had been married to her husband, José, for twelve years. José was a prominent physician. Rosa told me her husband's career was deeply important to him, and she sensed that she was not; José paid little attention to her.

Rosa was not passive or unaware of her feelings. She told her husband how unhappy she was and what she needed. He would seem to listen—and then simply ignore her concerns. He had done this from the beginning of their marriage.

I told Rosa that it was very helpful that she was aware of her own emotions. Yet it was clear to me she was also steeped in all the myths and principles of EN. These kept her feeling like a victim of her husband.

In therapy, she began to look at her EN, how fully she had embraced it, and how unhappy it had made her. She made a decision to live a different life.

Rosa realized she had married her husband because her mother, Nina, had strongly encouraged her to. Nina thought it would be great for her daughter to be married to a doctor. Looking back, Rosa wasn't even sure that, on her own, she would have chosen José as her husband.

Over time, Rosa began to listen to her own wisdom. She decided to separate from José for six months and see what happened. Soon her anger began to subside as she started to let go of EN. After nine months, she was able to go off the antidepressants, which she had been on for ten years.

Yet, at first, she was afraid to tell her mother, who lived on the west coast, about the separation. I encouraged her to accept the fear and tell her mother anyway—though I warned her that her mother would probably use the myths of EN to try to shame her.

That's exactly what happened. Rosa's mother said to her, multiple times, "I can't believe you separated from José! Don't you know how much that hurts your father and me?" Not once did Nina express any concern for Rosa, or ask about why she had made her choice, or try to learn how she was doing.

Rosa and José eventually got back together. José became much more respectful toward Rosa and more concerned about her feelings and needs. He also learned how to genuinely listen. For her part, Rosa learned how to step out of EN, take care of herself, and set boundaries. As a result, she realized that she now *wanted* to be married to José.

To our repeated shock and disappointment, EN doesn't make us safe or happy. Furthermore, people don't give us what we want. In fact, often they take from us and want or expect more. As Rosa did, we imagine that EN will eventually pay off. Yet it never does.

We start to get angry that others aren't paying attention to us or giving us what matters to us. We lived by Myths 1, 3, 4, and 5 and took care of them; why aren't they living by Myth 2 and taking care of us in return? We start to feel resentful.

Over time, these resentments build. And, either out loud or to ourselves, we say, "After all I've done for you, the least you could do for me is . . . " or "All I want for you to do is to . . . ; is that so much to ask?" We become martyrs.

> . . . we imagine that EN will eventually pay off.
> Yet it never does.

Here is what's actually happening: We want others to respect our desires, yet we don't respect our own. We want others to treat us as important, yet we don't treat *ourselves* as important.

At the same time, it feels frightening to stop pleasing others, stand up for ourselves, give ourselves what we want or need, and tell others clearly what we want from them. We know they might not say yes or give us what we want. Worse, they might also reject us, tell us we're selfish and bad, and then leave us.

## Trusting Your Feelings

Emotions are the language of the body. They are never wrong; they simply are. They arise, sometimes unexpectedly, and then you can recognize them, acknowledge them, and choose what to do about them. This is both a privilege and a responsibility.

Have you ever been told, "You're overly emotional" or "You're too sensitive"? Often this translates to, *I'm uncomfortable with the feelings you're expressing. I don't know how to take care of my own feelings, let alone yours. I'm caught up in Myth 2, so I expect you to take care of me and make me feel comfortable by no longer expressing your own feelings. Because of my EN, I never learned how to manage my emotions, so I need you to help manage them for me. Please don't express yourself authentically.*

Notice that this statement says everything about the speaker and little about you. (In any case, I've always wondered how people measure being "overly emotional." That scale seems to vary from one anxious, critical person to another.)

Our natural response to such phrases is to feel judged and rejected. If we hear words such as these over and over, we begin to imagine that the feelings that arise naturally in us must be wrong in some way. Eventually we may stop trusting our own emotions.

Such criticisms are difficult and painful enough when they occur between adults; however, they are even more painful when adults give them to kids. And when most of us were kids, such phrases were repeatedly said to us. Our parents, and other important adults in our life, taught us that there is something wrong with strong or painful emotions in general, or certain feelings in particular. Because other people felt uncomfortable when we expressed these feelings around them, they told us that *we* were wrong or bad to express those emotions—or even to experience them at all.

In practice, girls and women are often taught that they're too sensitive; that they let their feelings get hurt too easily; and that they "shouldn't" feel so hurt or frightened or worried. As they continue to hear these messages for years, they start doubting their own feelings.

Meanwhile, boys and men are often taught that feeling most of their emotions is wrong—yet feeling and expressing anger is okay. They're told that real men don't feel hurt, afraid, insecure, weak, or doubtful. And, over the years, they too begin to doubt, and sometimes fear, their own emotions—except for anger.

Actually, because of their EN, people regularly send each other similar messages. These are about more than just how they express their emotions: *You're too sloppy. You're too neat. You're too assertive. You're too passive. You talk on the phone too much. You don't answer your phone enough. You're too wishy-washy. You're too opinionated. You're too uncertain. You're too moderate.*

Often, these statements translate into the same message: *I'm uncomfortable with who you are and what you're doing. I'm caught up in Myth 2, so I expect you to take care of me and make me feel comfortable. Please don't be who you are or do what you're doing. Above all, please don't be authentic. Instead, I need you to act in ways that feel safe and familiar to me.*

## MARION AND HER MOTHER

When Marion is five years old, her mother accidently slams the car door on her fingers. Marion screams and starts crying. Her mother quickly opens the door and says, "Honey, I'm so sorry! Let me see your hand." She tries to take her daughter's hand; she can't, though, because Marion is jumping up and down in pain and shaking her arm and crying hysterically.

Her mom wasn't distracted or thoughtless when she closed the door on her daughter's hand. The injury was clearly an accident. Even five-year-old Marion understands this. And her mom understands that it is natural for her daughter to scream and jump up and down after her hand has been caught in a door.

Nevertheless, after Marion has screamed and jumped around for a time, her mother says to her, "Honey, I need you to stop crying right now. I hate to see you in such pain, and I'm starting to get very upset."

Marion immediately complies, for she knows from hard experience that she will face disapproval from her mom if she doesn't.

This and many other similar experiences teach Marion that she doesn't count; however, her mom does. If Marion doesn't take care of her mother's feelings, she will face shame, anger, rejection, or even all three.

It's important to repeat that one or two such incidents rarely do any lasting harm to kids. However, when similar events are repeated over and over—especially with children, who have very limited abilities to reason—they usually help EN to take root.

## AMELIA AND HER MOTHER

Amelia is the daughter of a Baptist minister. Growing up, Amelia attended church almost every Sunday. When she was in college, however, she became less and less interested in religion and eventually stopped going to church. She's not against religion or the Baptist faith; she simply no longer finds meaning in traditional church services, as she used to when she was growing up.

On Amelia's first weekend back home after her college graduation, her mother takes her aside and says, "Will you come to church with us on Sunday? It would make your father very happy."

"Thanks, Mom," Amelia says. "I appreciate the invite. On Sunday morning, though, I have a brunch date with some friends."

Her mother leans in closer. Almost whispering, she says, "Honey, I need to tell you something. Your daddy is very upset that you and your brother stopped going to church. He says he feels like a failure as a minister because of it. If you don't come on Sunday, everyone will ask about you, and I won't know what to tell them. I'll be so embarrassed. Come with us this Sunday and make both of us proud."

Amelia's story contains an entire cluster of boundary violations, all intertwined with the myths and principles of EN:

- Amelia's mother holds her responsible for how her father feels about himself as a minister.

- Her mother clearly believes that Ameila is responsible for making them happy on Sunday, and that Amelia will be responsible for embarrassing her if she doesn't show up at church.

- Amelia's mom also believes that her and her husband's concerns are more important than Amelia's. In fact, Amelia's mother never asks her daughter why she stopped going to church or what her current spiritual leanings are. Amelia's needs and concerns don't matter much to her mom.

- Her mom doesn't consider the potential disappointment or loss for Amelia and her friends if Amelia breaks her brunch date.

Amelia feels angry and discounted by her mom's request. However, she is aware enough to take a deep breath and say, "I made the brunch date three weeks ago—and I haven't seen my friends back home in months. I don't have plans for a week from Sunday, though, and there are people at church who I'd be happy to see again. I can come with you and Daddy then."

In making this decision, Amelia sets a clear and loving boundary with her parents. She lets her mom know that she cares about the family—and that she also cares about her friends and keeping an existing commitment to them. Furthermore, she makes it clear that she is not going to church the following Sunday to appease her parents or make them happy; she's doing it to renew some of her own relationships with other congregants.

Because of our EN, most of us also have a limited ability to know and communicate our emotional needs. We may experience sensations in our body, yet we usually don't examine them to discover what they are and what they are telling us. Instead, we disconnect from our body, go numb, and follow the myths of EN.

Because we often don't attend to what is going on inside us, we often say *I feel* and then add *that* or *like*:

- I feel that you were being thoughtless.
- I feel like what you're saying is wrong.
- I feel that it's too expensive.
- I feel that our country lets in too many immigrants.
- I feel like you haven't been listening to me.

However, whenever *I feel* is followed by *that* or *like*, what follows is *not* an emotion or physical sensation. It's actually a thought.

> Your emotions give you important information about who you are, what is going on for you, and what to do next.

Because we often say *I feel*, most of us think that when we use the phrase, we are communicating about our emotions. Yet we usually aren't. We are sharing our thoughts. We are often blaming someone or being critical. Meanwhile, we remain unaware of our own underlying feelings. And because of our blame or criticism, the person we're speaking with may become defensive, and genuine communication may come to a halt.

No matter what others may tell you or demand of you, feeling and trusting whatever emotion you experience is essential to your healing and your happiness. Your emotions give you important information about who you are, what is going on for you, and what to do next.

Trusting your emotions does *not* mean following any impulse that arises—or believing that feelings need to always overrule your experience, reason, or judgment. It simply means accepting each feeling as real, genuine, and valid; not doubting its legitimacy as an experience; and not denying, dismissing, or devaluing it.

All of this takes practice. Over time, however, as you the repeat the practices in this book, you will discover the wisdom of your emotions and the value of the information they provide.

## ASHA AND HER PARENTS

Asha is the youngest of four children. She has a sister who is four years older, and a brother and an adopted sister who are both two years older. Her family lives in a small town in Oregon.

Throughout her life, Asha has always had to share a room with one of her sisters. Then, when Asha is sixteen years old, her brother joins the Marines and her younger sister goes off to college. Asha is very excited for two reasons: she will have her own room for the first time and she will be the only child at home. She hopes that, for the first time in her life, she will get to feel special, have her parents' full attention, and be regularly listened to. She intuitively knows how critical this time is for her.

Asha has never felt a strong connection with her parents, both of whom work long hours at the bookkeeping firm they own. Now that all her siblings are gone, Asha hopes that she and her parents will have a chance to grow closer.

Two weeks after her sister leaves for college, Asha's parents get a call from the local sheriff. The sheriff explains he has a sixteen-year-old girl in lockup. Hallie ran away from her aunt's home in Minnesota, and before that she had a long history of running away from foster homes. A judge gave her one last chance to avoid being sent to a juvenile detention center by staying with her aunt.

Hallie will go to a court hearing in two weeks. The sheriff, who does not want to keep Hallie in jail with adult criminals, knows that Asha's parents have a reputation for helping kids at risk. He asks them if Hallie can stay with them for two weeks. They agree.

Asha wishes her parents had checked with her before saying yes. Still, she is not terribly hurt or concerned, because Hallie will only be staying with her family for two weeks.

When Hallie arrives, Asha treats her respectfully. Hallie responds in kind, and Asha begins mentally counting down the days until she leaves.

At the court hearing, which Asha's parents attend while she is at school, the judge tells Hallie that he is sending her to juvenile detention. Hallie begins to cry. Then Asha's parents stand up and suggest to the judge that she allow Hallie to stay with them as a foster child until she turns eighteen. The judge agrees to consider this.

A few days later, Asha's parents get a phone call from the judge's office, letting them know that he has approved the foster care arrangement.

That evening, Asha's parents tell her the news. She feels crushed. Her hopes, dreams, and plans have been dashed. What hurts her still more, though, is that her parents made the decision without even checking with her.

For years, Asha has sensed that her parents saw her, the youngest child, as unimportant, a mere afterthought in the family. She hoped that would finally change. Instead, her parents ignored her and her desires once again. For Asha this is an old, familiar, and painful experience.

Asha has the courage to not passively accept this boundary violation. That night, after Hallie is asleep, she goes to her parents' bedroom and asks them, "Why couldn't you talk to me about Hallie before you decided?"

Her parents look at each other. Then her mother says, "Asha! You wouldn't want Hallie to be locked up, would you?"

Asha starts to cry. Yet she still has the presence of mind to say, "I am *not* sharing a room with her. And next time you have to make an important decision that involves me, talk to me about it first. Otherwise, *I* might be the one who runs away!"

Asha's final sentence is over-the-top teenage bluster. However, the rest of what she says is quite wise. She is honoring herself and her feelings and setting a clear boundary with her parents.

## What You Want

An important part of honoring your truth is having—and working to achieve—your own goals and dreams.

Many of us were taught to ignore or set aside our dreams and desires—or to not have dreams or desires at all—and, instead, to assist others in achieving what *they* desire or dream of. Too many of us try to find vicarious meaning through helping our partner or child achieve their dreams, while abandoning our own.

---

## HEALING ACTIVITY #8

### Explore Your Personal Desires

To help you get back in touch with what you care about, what holds meaning for you, and what you hope for and dream of, in your healing notebook write a list of at least fifteen things you want *for yourself*. Not for your kids. Not for your parents. Not for others you care about. Not for the world. For *you* and you alone.

Please dream big here. Don't let your concerns about age, money, education, or time get in your way. Remember, right now you're *dreaming*, not *planning*. However, don't list things that are outright impossible, such as *I want to be ten years younger* or *I want to be a World War II war hero*.

Each item needs to be specific. For example:

- I want to join a golf club this year.
- I want to go to Italy for two weeks before I turn forty.
- I want to resume my monthly lunches with Elaine.
- I want to spend two hours each week learning to draw (or meditate, or sing gospel, or cook Greek food).

List only things that energize you and make you happy whenever you do them, and whenever you simply think about doing them. So don't list goals such as *I want to lose twenty pounds* or *I want to find a better job*. Those may be worthy enough goals; however, they don't touch your heart or bring you joy and excitement the way dreams do.

Take as much time as you need to look into your own heart and create this list. If it takes you several days to mull over your options and assemble an honest and thoughtful list, that's fine. For many people with EN, it may take weeks or months to get started.

Once you've written this list, date it and post it in a place where you can see it regularly.

In the pages to come, you'll discover a process to begin turning the items on this list into things you actually *do*.

This list is not meant to be static. It's an ongoing process. The point is not to finish the list. In fact, once you've started to work seriously on one, please add a new one, so you always have at least fifteen things on your list. This will help you maintain a habit of identifying, imagining, and doing things that bring you pleasure or joy.

Eventually, as your life unfolds and you do more and more of the things on this list, going after your dreams will come naturally.

# 5

# How Rules Help Us
# and Harm Us

"When you begin to touch your heart or let your
heart be touched, you begin to discover that it's
bottomless, that it doesn't have any resolution,
that this heart is huge, vast, limitless. You begin
to discover how much warmth and gentleness are
there, as well as how much space."

*Pema Chödrön*

Until the age of five, most us expressed our thoughts, feelings, and
needs with little regard to whether they helped us to belong. This
expression was as natural to us as breathing. We intuitively sensed
who we were, what we wanted, how we felt, what we liked, and what
we disliked. We were intimately familiar with our bodies and our
boundaries—our truths.

A four-year-old boy comes over to visit his friend from daycare. The visitor picks up a toy truck. It's the other boy's favorite truck, so he screams and hits his friend.

When a three-year-old girl asks her equally young friend if she can give him a hug, he clearly says, "No!"

When a father asks his two-year-old daughter if she wants some sweet potatoes, she shakes her head and says, "No."

All of this free and authentic expression creates chaos. The more children, the more chaos. Anyone who interacts with small kids knows this.

We have a paradox here: on the one hand, parents need to devise clear, simple rules for their kids in order to limit chaos. On the other hand, parents also have to understand enough about child development that they don't ask their kids to do the impossible.

Parents often try to teach children under the age of five some rules about sharing, asking for what they want, and not screaming, grabbing, or hitting people. However, *much of this unpleasant behavior is appropriate for kids that young.* They haven't yet developed the necessary self-control.

Before the age of three, kids normally don't share. They're simply unable to. Yet many parents insist on trying to teach the concept to very young children—some as young as six to nine months. Asking a two-year-old to share is like asking a seven-year-old to drive a car. Parallel play (kids playing separately, side by side) is normal for children under the age of three. Sharing is not.

Language development plays an integral role in building self-control, and this doesn't usually begin until around age five. Until then, although kids may parrot what they hear from adults, they don't comprehend the full meaning of the words they're repeating.

Most kids under the age of five do develop some limited and rudimentary self-control. If a moment is not highly emotionally charged for them, *some* self-control is possible. However, if something emotional occurs—such as a sibling grabbing a toy away—then the self-control typically flies out the window. This is partly what makes birthdays and holidays so challenging.

Furthermore, kids under the age of two-and-a-half or three also haven't developed the language ability to articulate their feelings, wants, or needs in a way that adults deem appropriate. (This varies somewhat from one child to another, of course.) As children, learning to articulate our feelings in a socially acceptable way takes years of learning and practice—and a lot of trial and error. And that's if we're fortunate enough to be encouraged to do so.

In practice, most of us are not taught—or encouraged, or permitted—to name our feelings and discuss them. Instead, we are taught to hide and ignore them. And in most cases, we eventually pass on this lesson to our own children. The result is that most very young children experience feeling rejected, excluded, or judged by adults for not knowing or following adult rules and expectations. Yet, often, those rules and expectations are not reasonable or realistic for people their age.

I often observe adults shaming young children for not behaving like ten-year-olds when they are only three or four or five. For example, in a restaurant, I watched the parents of a four-year-old girl berate her for not sitting quietly beside them for an hour while they talked and ate. This is like punishing your dog for not being a cat. When a child is three or four—or five, seven, or eight—they are *unable* to behave like a ten-year-old; they're developmentally too young. This is also why a child who is identified as gifted, and thus allowed to skip a grade, may become very anxious. Although they are able to handle the academics, they can't skip a year of social development. That goes at its own pace for everyone.

We parents often don't understand what is developmentally normal—or possible. As a result, our expectations are often unrealistically high, especially for firstborns. Then, through our own ignorance, we disapprove of our children—or get angry with them for doing something they didn't know they weren't supposed to do. This wounds the children, who then develop shame.

Sadly, this turns out to be the case with most parents and their children. Then, as those children become adults and have kids of their own, they set the same unrealistic expectations and pass on the same shame—while believing they're doing the right things for *their* children.

# CHELSEA AND MAGGIE AND THEIR GRANDMOTHER

Two-and-a-half-year-old Maggie and four-year-old Chelsea are playing house at their grandmother's home, having tea with her antique children's china set. The girls love to play with this special set of dishes.

Their grandmother Jenny has asked them to hold their tea party in the carpeted part of the living room, so that if either girl drops a dish, it will be much less likely to shatter. Several times she said to them, "Please keep the china away from the tile."

As Jenny watches from her desk across the room, however, the girls carry dishes across the house, walking across a three-foot strip of tile. She says sternly, "Remember what I said about the tile, girls!"

In the half hour that follows, Jenny sees both girls carry china across the tiled area multiple times. Finally she stands up and says, raising her voice, "You girls aren't listening to me. You're going to drop something on that tile floor!"

The girls turn and stare at her. Fortunately, because of their confused expressions, Jenny has the presence of mind to ask, "Excuse me, girls. Do either of you know what tile is?"

Both girls shake their heads.

Jenny smiles and says, "Well, then. Let me show you." She does, and the behavior that Jenny had become so vexed about immediately ceases. The girls keep their tea party in the carpeted area.

As Jenny watches her granddaughters from her desk a few minutes later, she reminds herself that children often know far less about the world than adults imagine they do.

Through EN, day by day and generation after generation, we repeat this message and reenact this pattern: *In order to be loved and accepted, children must learn to follow and conform to rules—both the helpful and the unhelpful ones.*

When we're young, our minds and hearts are largely incapable of telling the difference between the rules that help us survive and thrive, and the ones that wound us. Instead, most of us simply adhere to the rules, hoping that doing so will keep us physically and emotionally safe. Yet the more time and energy we expend trying to keep ourselves safe through our obedience, the more we lose touch with our true selves.

Some of us are intuitively aware of this insidious process, though we are too young to be able to articulate it to others, or even to ourselves. So, in response to the myths of EN—and in an attempt to keep a part of our true self alive—some of us rebel. We break many of the rules, both the pernicious rules surrounding EN *and* some rules that are genuinely helpful and protective.

*Both* of these responses—trying to protect ourselves by obeying all the rules *and* rebelling against many of the rules that adults make for us—ultimately prove inadequate for living a happy adult life.

As kids, most of us choose the first response. We learn to accept and follow rules, largely without questioning them. As a result, we slowly separate ourselves from our own truth, our own internal wisdom, our own experience, our own emotional needs, and the wisdom of our bodies and our authentic selves. We may stop listening to what our bodies tell us. Because we have learned to spend much of our time and energy taking care of others, day by day we further lose touch with ourselves.

By the age of fifteen, many of us are pretty much asleep—disconnected from ourselves. We have fully integrated the habit of obeying rules—and the myths and principles of EN—into our psyches.

Beginning at about the age of thirteen, if we're raised in a reasonably functional family, we turn to our peers rather than our parents for our greatest connections and directions. This is a big step toward our emancipation—and part of our healthy development. As part of this breaking away from our parents, we naturally start testing their values, challenging the rules, and expressing more of ourselves.

In doing so, we begin to learn what *we* believe and think, rather than merely taking on what we have been taught to believe. This is quite healthy, especially if we do it at an age where our parents are willing and able to be a safety net for us

If our parents instead punish us rather harshly or reject us for this normal "rebellion," we may turn primarily to our peers for our acceptance and love. We want to be seen, acknowledged, and valued for who we are and what we think and believe. During adolescence, our peers will often do that far more than our parents will. In fact, many parents, caught up in Myth 2, will feel very frightened and out of control as their kids go through adolescence and begin to have ideas and beliefs of their own.

Unfortunately, many of us are so steeped in our EN during this period that we don't go through either variation of this process. Instead, we stay compliant. We generally do what adults tell us to—and we mostly keep our mouths shut. As a result, our development is stunted.

## TOPHER AND HIS SCIENCE TEACHER

When Topher is thirteen, his family moves from Charlotte, North Carolina to Portland, Maine. At Topher's new middle school, the teachers and rules are much stricter than they were in North Carolina. Topher is surprised by the strictness at first. Soon he accepts it, though, and does his best to follow the rules and thus be considered good and lovable.

One of the rules in Topher's science class is that any assignment turned in late receives an automatic F. Another is that each student is allowed to be late for class a total of three times each semester; if a student is late four times, his or her final grade for the course is lowered by one letter.

One afternoon, before the bell rings, Topher's science teacher begins to collect the homework from the night before. Topher suddenly realizes that he left his assignment in his locker, so he asks the teacher if he can take one of his tardies and go get his homework. The teacher says, "Okay. Your assignment will still be late, though, since you won't have it in the room by the time the bell rings. So you'll still get an F."

The structure the teacher set up about assignments being on time is both reasonable and helpful. It teaches students to be responsible. However, the teacher's rigidity in this case doesn't help Topher to be more responsible. Instead, it teaches him that following a rule is more important than the people the rule is meant to serve.

Topher says, "Never mind," takes the F, and leaves his homework in his locker.

From this interaction, Topher learns that the rules in his science class are more important than him or his education. This leaves him feeling temporarily worthless and discouraged. He is trying his best to do things right, and his intentions are honorable. Furthermore, this is the first time he's forgotten his homework, and he hasn't even left it at home. It's only a one-minute walk away.

The same thing happens again two months later. This time, when Topher realizes he has left his homework in his locker, he doesn't even bother saying anything. When the teacher asks him where his homework is, he just shrugs.

The two Fs drag down Topher's final grade from a B+ to a C+. He becomes discouraged and feels hopeless, powerless, and misunderstood. His enthusiasm for trying to get good grades wanes.

....................................................................................................

As more years pass, most of us become less and less conscious of our true selves. We move further and further away from listening to and caring for our own needs and wants. Instead of attending to our own wisdom, we allow our old wounds—the wounds of not being important, counted, or likeable—to be repeatedly reinjured. Tragically, by the time we are adults, we learn to deepen these wounds by calling *ourselves* stupid, lazy, hopeless, or a loser—all in attempt to get ourselves to shape up and not make a painful mistake again.

For many of us, the resulting trauma becomes too much to endure. So we attempt to mask or avoid the pain through drug and alcohol abuse, harmful sexual behavior, perfectionism, workaholism, compulsive eating, or other hurtful activities.

## The Benefits and Drawbacks of Rules

Around the age of five, most of us enter the larger world outside of home and daycare. This is the world of school, the neighborhood, a religious community or institution, organized sports, and training in dance, music, or some other art. As our world expands, we learn there are more and more rules to know and follow. As we learn these rules, the chaos in our lives starts to diminish.

Five and six year olds love rules, and love to tell others when they are not following rules. This is how kids' socialization begins in earnest. For kids at this age, habits, schedules, rules, and other forms of structure help to make the world predictable. They also help children feel safe and secure. Kids begin to know what to do and what not to do and can count on the rules to remove or reduce uncertainty and chaos.

Rules are also a sign of caring. One of my clients told me that when he was in elementary school, his parents let him ride his bike in the evening as late as he wanted. His friends thought he was lucky because he could stay out late. However, he didn't feel lucky. He told me, "I wish they'd called me in for bed. It would have been a sign that they cared."

However, not all rules, or all forms of their enforcement, are helpful. When a rule becomes inflexible, or more important than the people it is meant to serve, rigidity sets in and people get wounded. When a rule doesn't serve the relevant people, it usually needs to be altered, not enforced with greater fervor.

For example, imagine you are hosting a slumber party for your daughter's ninth birthday. Her regular bedtime of 8:30 p.m. is reasonable on most nights. However, enforcing it at the slumber party would disappoint her and her friends. This would be a good night to make an exception and change her bedtime to 10:00 or 10:30 p.m., which would make the party feel special.

When adults judge, shame, or reject their kids for not following rules—even when the rules are helpful—they unwittingly promote the development of EN. This is especially true when adults make it clear that following a rule is more important than caring for or being of service to human beings.

And, of course, some rules simply don't serve anyone. Yet we often adopt them without testing their accuracy, measuring their value, or considering their potential harm.

Many of these rules begin as aphorisms or sayings. Here are some common examples:

- "Children should be seen and not heard."
- "Keep your feelings to yourself."
- "Boys who cry or get scared are sissies."
- "To be emotional is to be weak."
- "Real men don't cry."
- "Women who are assertive are bitchy."
- "'Tis better to give than to receive."
- "It's important to tell white lies, so as not to not hurt others."
- "Taking time for yourself is selfish."

Rather than creating order, many of these rules only create wounds.

As you learn more about EN, you may find yourself evaluating your own parenting, as well as the rules you use with your children and teach to them. This process of self-evaluation can be beneficial—and potentially enlightening. However, it's important to remember that healing your own EN wounds and being a loving parent go hand-in-hand. As you heal, you will automatically become a better and more compassionate mom or dad.

> . . . healing your own EN wounds and being
> a loving parent go hand-in-hand.

So be compassionate with yourself as well. If you see that you are acting out of your own unhealed childhood wounds, don't shame yourself or tell yourself that you've been a bad parent. This won't benefit you *or* your kids. Instead, use this knowledge to bring more compassion to yourself—and to how hard you are trying to do a good job as a mother or father. Remind yourself that you are wounded and traumatized—and doing your best. Be gentle with yourself.

None of us is a perfect parent. Most of us, including most of us therapists, routinely fall far short of that ideal. As you heal your old wounds, your own parenting (and grandparenting) will improve greatly, no matter how young or old your children or grandchildren are. In turn, this will help your children's wounds begin to heal as well.

Now it's time for you to examine and challenge some of the rules you learned as a child. As you will discover, this is a profound act of healing and self-love.

In the chapters that follow, you will continue to:

- Explore more of the rules you were taught as a child.
- Evaluate which rules make sense, which need to be adapted, and which to drop.
- Create new rules that can enrich your life.

Remember, no one else can do this for you. This is your own unique journey—a journey back to your true self. This journey will often be unsettling and, at times, even frightening. However, as you will see, it will also be exciting—and its rewards will be immeasurable.

# Lying to Survive

"As soon as you trust yourself,
you will know how to live."

*Johann Wolfgang von Goethe*

At a very young age, most of us are taught to lie by our families, our schools, our religious institutions, and society at large. We are not merely taught the behavior; we are also taught that lying is the correct and proper way to get through life. This is primarily taught to us through the principles of EN, and through Myths 1 and 5.

Over time, as these myths and principles become embedded in us, we systematically learn to be liars. Even though we're directly told lying is wrong, we're also taught, through what we see and experience, that we need to lie in order to belong.

As we've already seen, most of us learn to pretend to be different from who we actually are. We do this in order to fit in, feel safe, and survive. This is itself a form of ongoing lying.

We are also trained to lie in other ways. In fact, in our culture, lying is both encouraged and considered normal: *Tell Grandma how glad you are to see her. And remember, look surprised and happy when she gives you one of her fruitcakes.* Indeed, in some contexts, lying is often valued more than the truth: *I told her I really liked her new dress because I didn't want to hurt her feelings. Doesn't she look awful in it, though?*

Our first lessons in learning to lie about who we are usually occur in our family. This is true even if our parents are good people who have the best of intentions.

Although most children hear their parents talk about the importance of being honest, they frequently hear them lie. They hear their parents express one opinion to their friends or relatives and the opposite opinion to each other. They hear their parents lie to strangers about their ages, about being busy when they are not, and about their feelings. Their parents may pretend to outsiders that everyone in the family is happy, even though there may be physical abuse or addiction or a child who is failing in school.

As kids, most of us also heard our parents lie to each other. And it's not uncommon for one parent to ask a child to lie to the other parent: *Don't tell your father we went to the movies; he'll just get angry.*

We also learn to lie through omission. Although we don't tell a direct lie with words, we leave out important information. For example, your teenage daughter admits to you that there was some drinking at the party she attended. However, she doesn't tell you about the drugs she was offered or that the parents weren't home.

By the time most of us turn eight or nine, we've caught our parents lying to us multiple times. And being lied to always wounds us.

To children, every broken promise may be experienced as a lie, even when one is broken for the best of reasons. When a mother says to her daughter, "I know I promised we'd go to the beach today, honey. Your brother's sick, though, so I need to take him to the doctor." Even though mom is doing the responsible thing, her daughter still feels disappointed and, perhaps, angry and betrayed. The daughter is wounded because her mother broke a promise to her. Her wound is unavoidable, yet it is real.

Many parents also train their children to lie for them: *If someone calls, tell them I'm at the office. Then come and tell me who it was.*

Eventually we learn that lying is both common and acceptable.

Myth 1 further encourages us to lie. In following it, we learn to lie to others—*Your broccoli and cheese casserole was delicious*—instead of learning to tell the truth graciously—*Thank you for having me over for dinner; I appreciate the time and care you took in preparing it, and I had a lovely evening.*

Most of us get further lessons in lying at school. We learn at a very young age not to say, "Teacher, I'm lost," because at some point a teacher called us stupid or inattentive. We learn not to tell our teachers that something is dull or confusing because we know they may shame us in response. We learn that correcting a teacher who makes an error may get us sent to the principal's office. This is why some kids go through school never asking questions, never raising their hand, and saying as little as possible. It is also the exact opposite of expressing their truths. And it is another example of the lie of omission.

> True caring always involves the other person's wishes and needs *and* our own.

Our religious institutions encourage lying as well. When we're kids, these institutions make it clear to us that when they ask us for something—to help out at a worship service, go on a group camping trip, or collect money from our parents—it's not okay to say, "No, thank you; I'm not interested." We either need to treat the request as an order and say yes or lie about our reason for saying no: *I already promised my sister I'd take her skating that morning. I'll be on vacation that Sunday. We'll be visiting my grandparents in Ohio.*

Many of us have also been taught by our religion that taking care of our own needs is selfish and unspiritual. Of course, unbridled hedonism or extreme self-indulgence aren't good for anyone. However, in a world we share with others, it's never a matter of taking care of others *or* taking care of ourselves. True caring always involves the other person's wishes and needs *and* our own.

Yet we're often taught to be selfless, even at our own—and others'—peril. For instance, we're taught to always agree to volunteer for a good cause, even when we're sick and want to say no. So we help out, resent every minute of it, infect half the volunteers we work with, and get sicker ourselves. Everyone would have been better off if we'd just stayed home.

Often, when we consider others' needs and ignore our own, this is a form of manipulation: we're trying to impress others with how kind or caring or capable we are, so they will like us. Psychologist Sondra Smalley calls this *impression management*.

Religious institutions teach us to lie in still other ways. We're taught to deny our sexuality; to never express our anger, because to do so would be unspiritual or un-Christ-like; to not challenge spiritual leaders on their questionable or unacceptable behavior; or to "just believe" or "just have faith," when we actually don't.

As we age, society at large also teaches us to lie. We learn that governments—both large and small—and political leaders lie to us (e.g., the Watergate and Iran-Contra scandals); financial institutions lie to us (e.g., the financial collapse in 2007 and 2008); other kinds of corporations lie to us; religious institutions lie to us; and the media lie to us. Eventually we come to accept this behavior as normal—the way things are—and we come to expect it.

As a result of all this, not being honest about who we are, what we feel, what we want and don't want, and what we stand for is also considered normal. However, there is a huge cost to this: we end up not honoring or valuing ourselves—and not knowing who we are.

Worse still, because most of us have our own pattern of lying, we often don't trust what others say to us. We assume they are lying as well. This is true even if we care deeply about them, and they care deeply about us. Think of all the times you've questioned something your partner or good friend said, even though they were perfectly clear: *Are you sure you're okay with that? Really? Are you sure you're not mad? You feel the same way I do?*

We simply don't trust others. Because we routinely lie, and because we have heard others lie, we assume that others routinely lie to us as well. And, given how much people lie to one another, why would we think otherwise?

## Lying to Ourselves

Most of us also learn to lie to ourselves, primarily through denial. We deny what we observe or feel and replace those observations or feelings with the myths and principles of EN. We also tell ourselves that making someone else feel good is more important than expressing our truth or living according to our values.

As children, denial is often a necessary survival tool because the truth is often too unbearable for us to live with, and we don't have the power to change our situation. So we either sit inside our pain or, much more commonly, deny it by learning to shut down our heart and distract ourselves. We immerse ourselves in books, throw ourselves into social media, watch TV, play video games, or look at YouTube videos. All of these activities help us go numb and avoid some of the pain. Meanwhile, we deny our own truth—and continue to lose touch with who we truly are.

As we grow up, we typically gain some power to change our situation. However, by then our denial of pain and difficulty may have become a habit. We fall back into denial because we're used to it, and because it was the best and most effective tool we had when we were young.

> As children, denial is often a necessary survival tool because the truth is often too unbearable for us to live with, and we don't have the power to change our situation.

Even though more effective responses are now available to us, we stick with what we're used to. Even when we have the power to modify our situation (or ourselves), often we don't. Instead, when we experience deep pain, we try to distract ourselves from it with alcohol or other drugs, overworking, affairs, etc. Denial thus becomes one of the primary ways we harm ourselves as adults.

We practice denial in relation to our emotions when we tell ourselves things such as *It really wasn't that big a deal*; or, *She didn't mean to hurt me*; or, *I'm being overly sensitive*; or, *He couldn't help it*.

We also deny how we feel physically and push ourselves when we are exhausted. We go to work when we are sick. We don't seek medical advice when we need to.

We deny what we want or need: *It means a lot to my wife if we go here to eat; maybe next time we can go someplace else.* Or, *My boss really needs me to work late; I'll mow the lawn tomorrow night.* A problem occurs when we consider *only* the other person's wishes and deny our own.

In addition, we deny what we observe or know to be true in other people: *He's a teenage boy; he'll grow out of it.* Or, *My husband threatened me because he had a very tough week at work; he'll be okay in the morning. If I make his favorite breakfast, he'll treat me the way he used to.*

We believe—incorrectly—that the truth is too painful to face. We think we'll die or go crazy if we admit that our partner is an alcoholic; our daughter has a serious eating disorder; our relationship with our children is fraught with conflict and pain; or our partner is having an affair. We imagine that we cannot handle the truth, so instead we live in a fantasy of how we wish things could be.

An important first step in healing from everyday narcissism is letting go of the habit of lying— first to yourself, then to others.

We imagine—also incorrectly—that all of this denial allows us to avoid the pain of what is. We also use our denial as an excuse to do nothing to change our situation (or ourselves). All of this denial of our situation also requires us to deny our own feelings, wants, and needs.

The more we lie to ourselves or stay in denial, the less we are able to heal, move forward, and create the life we long for. And the more we lie or deny things to ourselves, the further we get from our true self. Honesty with ourselves thus becomes our greatest challenge—and our deepest need.

An important first step in healing from everyday narcissism is letting go of the habit of lying—first to yourself, then to others. In the activities that follow, you'll begin to practice being honest with yourself. As this becomes a habit, you'll also practice being honest with others.

## HEALING ACTIVITY #9

### Speak Your Truth

Begin to practice speaking your truth in a loving and respectful way, whenever and wherever you are. The key here is *a loving and respectful way*. If your partner makes a reasonable request, such as *Please help me clear the table*, and you don't want to, it's neither loving nor respectful to say, "No. Leave me alone," or "Forget it; I'm not in the mood." It's also unloving and disrespectful to simply ignore their request.

Instead, you might say, "I'm really tired, yet I know you spent a long time cooking lunch, so, yes, of course," or "I need to lie down for a bit, so if you leave the dishes, I'll take care of them when I get up." In either case, you speak your truth and respect yourself, while also respecting your partner and accepting the demands of the situation.

When someone asks you to do something you don't want to do, simply say, "No, that won't work for me," or "No, I don't want to," or just "No." If they push you to change your mind, just smile and say no again. When we make excuses—which are sometimes lies—we give our power away because we're attempting to get the other person's permission to say no. We tell ourselves that if we can obtain this permission, the person won't be mad at us and reject us. However, as adults we don't need permission to be true to ourselves. (Of course, don't use this as an excuse to be thoughtless or disrespectful—or to avoid a genuine responsibility, such as keeping an appointment or picking up your child at school.)

Saying a simple "No," or "No, that won't work for me," creates a firm, clear boundary between you and the other person. Sometimes this kind of boundary—a barrier, really— is exactly what you want and need.

For example, if someone you are not interested in dating keeps asking you out, then a simple "No" (or "No, I'm not interested," or even "No, and please stop asking") is probably the best answer. If you say "No, not this weekend," or "Not when I'm so busy at work," or "Not while my kids are still in school," you leave the door open for the future, and the person will likely keep coming back.

Now let's flip this over. If you *do* want to leave a door open, then clearly do so; don't say "No, thank you" or "Nope, not for me." Add a qualifier and a potential connection or opportunity: "No, this weekend won't work for me. Let's find another time to get together." You are creating a connection instead of a barrier.

In either case you are clearly and straightforwardly speaking your truth.

Too often, many of us say yes to a request without considering how it feels. Later, we may wish we hadn't agreed. With this in mind, please practice not responding to requests immediately. Instead, say, "Let me think about it. I'll get back to you in ____ minutes/hours/days." Take the time to check in with your body and listen to your own truth. Then, based on your body's reaction and your own careful consideration, speak your truth to the person who made the request.

Here are some other ways to practice speaking your truth:

· Next time you realize that you are lying, either to someone else or to yourself, pay attention to how it feels in your body. Most of the time, you'll get a signal that tells you something is not okay.

· Each day, keep track of how many times you didn't speak your truth or act truthfully. With each new day that passes, try to reduce that number.

· Each time you speak your truth, pay attention to how it feels in your body. It may feel scary at first. It will also feel empowering.

Sometimes you may feel two different, or even contradictory, truths at once. For example, imagine you come home exhausted from work. You have already committed to attending a meeting at your child's school that evening. Your body tells you that you need rest; yet your brain and heart tell you that you want to support your daughter by meeting with her and her teacher. *Each of these impulses reflects one of your truths.*

Here's what's so empowering: choosing *either one* enables you to honor yourself and your truth. The actual choice you make will depend on your priorities and the specifics of the situation. For example, do you have to get up early tomorrow, or can you sleep in? Can you plan to meet privately with your child's teacher and skip the meeting with all the other parents? Is your daughter seven or seventeen?

However, going out dancing with your partner when you're exhausted because your partner is feeling bored and lonely does *not* honor you. If you catch yourself thinking, *If I do that, it will mean I'm a really selfish person*, examine that thought carefully. Is it an accurate assessment of the situation and your motives, or is one of the internalized EN myths speaking?

Keep in mind that it is usually possible to care for yourself *and* someone else; most situations are not either/or. Furthermore, you can have conflicting wants or impulses and still remain a caring person.

At other times, your truth may conflict with the truth of someone else you care about. This conflict doesn't have to be a problem. If the two of you are willing to let go of the EN myths, speak your truths to each other with kindness, and listen with full attention and caring, you will often find a way to honor both people's truths. At the very least, you will be able to honor each other's boundaries.

## Speaking Difficult Truths

Some truths are far easier to express than others—and some people are easier to tell the truth to than others.

For some of us, being truthful with the people we're close to is much easier than speaking our truth to people we don't know well. For others, it's far easier to tell the truth to strangers and casual acquaintances. And for still other people, being fully honest with anyone seems impossible—or terrifying. As Ralph Waldo Emerson wrote in his essay "Self-Reliance," "Speak what you think now in hard words and to-morrow speak what to-morrow thinks in hard words[2] again, though it contradict every thing you said today." In doing so we begin to know what we really think and feel.

---

## HEALING ACTIVITY #10

---

### Clarify Your Truth

Most of the time, in speaking your truth out loud, you will know almost immediately, and without equivocation, whether you are expressing that truth fully and accurately. You'll say something out loud, notice how it feels in your body, and know if it's what you were really trying to say. At times you will realize that it wasn't exactly what you meant. That's when it's important to say, "No that's not quite right; let me try again," or "Wait, that's not the right word." You can then voice your thoughts and feelings until the words feel correct. Your body will let you know when what you've said matches what you mean.

It's important to practice this process. Keeping ideas and feelings locked inside, even if you review them carefully in your head, will not give you the same clarity you'll achieve by saying them out loud.

Expressing your thoughts and emotions aloud is like going shopping for a jacket: you wouldn't buy one without trying it on. When you do try it on, you know immediately if it fits, if it's comfortable, and if you like the style. Saying something out loud does the exact same thing for your feelings and thoughts.

---

2    Or, as we would say today, say it strongly, as if you mean it.

An essential part of speaking your truth is knowing that you don't have to say it perfectly the first time. You have a right to change your words, and even change your mind, in order to get closer to your truth.

It is often tempting to try to soften a difficult truth with qualifiers such as "sometimes," "a little," "kind of," "sort of," "maybe," "perhaps," and so on. We hope that by adding these words, other people will more readily accept what we have to say and not get angry or hurt. We especially hope they will still like us and not go away.

In using these qualifiers, though, we don't fully own what we are saying. We avoid declaring our whole truth and being true selves—all out of a fear of being rejected. So stop using qualifiers unless you genuinely want to qualify something. Just speak your truth. You will discover that it is both empowering and delightful to speak from your authentic self.

As Emerson noted, your truth may change—perhaps radically—as time passes, sometimes even in just a few minutes. As you grow, learn, and get new information, your viewpoint may change. This is normal, natural, and healthy.

As you will discover, speaking your truth is always empowering, even when people react badly to it. As Emerson also stated in "Self-Reliance," "Is it so bad then to be misunderstood? Pythagoras was misunderstood, and Socrates, and Jesus, and Luther, and Copernicus, and Galileo, and Newton, and every pure and wise spirit that ever took flesh."

Yes, speaking your truth will likely scare some people. You will not be very socially predictable. Others will see that you cannot be easily controlled or manipulated or made to feel guilty. Yet all of this will only make you feel more powerful—because you will *be* more powerful. Other people will experience you as more powerful as well. Some people will value this immensely; others will be put off or offended by it.

Speaking in this way can be very frightening at first, especially for women. Strong women who speak their truths are often called bitches or castrating females, particularly by frightened or angry men. Such name-calling is always a form of EN because it always carries this message: *when you tell the truth, you are not worthy, likeable, lovable, or desirable.* You'll recognize this as a version of Myth 5.

> ... speaking your truth will likely scare some people.

Too many women believe these false accusations and respond to them by backing down, keeping quiet, or relinquishing their power. In doing so, these women allow others (usually men) to control and define them.

---

### KAREN AND MARTY

Karen tells her husband, Marty, that she wants to see the movie *The Help*. He responds, "It's a stupid movie about some women who decided to go on strike. Why would you want to see that?" Karen, who has a PhD in chemistry, is surprised by her husband's strong reaction. She doesn't want him to see her as stupid, and she doesn't want to upset him or create conflict, so she lets the matter drop.

Imagine that Karen instead speaks her truth and honors herself by saying to Marty, "*The Help* is supposed to be very entertaining, with a good script, great acting, and an empowering message. Anyway, it's a film I want to see, no matter what my reasons are. Will you go with me?" Here are some of the things Marty might have said in response:

- "I didn't know the film had gotten good reviews. Sure, I'll see it with you, if next week we can see a movie that I pick."

- "Sorry, I'm not interested. Go see it with a friend sometime."

- "I didn't realize that seeing that particular movie was important to you. If that's really what you most want to see, I'll join you."

- "The plot sounded pretty stupid to me at first. So let me see what kind of a rating it got on Rotten Tomatoes . . . Wow, it got a 76 percent rating. Okay, I'll give it a try."

- "I still think it's stupid to want to see it. I'm not going."

If Marty's response is respectful (as it is in the first four responses) and Karen is acknowledged, then she and Marty have an honest and trusting interaction as a result. And even the final response, in which Marty is demeaning, offers Karen an opportunity to speak her truth; she can say, "Well, I feel differently. I'm going to see it with a friend."

Notice that both of these outcomes are better than Karen letting Marty bully her into silence and acquiescence.

As you speak your truth, again and again and again, your anger about life will steadily dissipate. You will begin to know yourself better—and enjoy life more.

When you speak your truth to your friends, some may find it difficult to hear or accept. A few may even go away as a result. This is most people's biggest fear when they first show their authentic selves. However, the friends who will stick around and stick by you will be your true friends because they will like you for who you truly are, not for whom you pretend to be.

Furthermore, when you speak your truth, some people will be grateful for your honesty and will trust and respect you even more. They may even thank you for being so honest. Because they can count on you to be truthful, they won't have to guess whether you really mean what you say. And almost nothing feels better than being in relationship with someone who cares for you, warts and all. Your honesty will also give others permission to be honest with you and share some of their own important truths with you. This will create more comfort, more safety, and more intimacy. You will also discover that the more you speak your truth, the easier it will be to do so next time.

It takes courage to speak our truth because doing so often feels like it threatens our ability to belong. We intuitively sense that we are not following the rules of EN. *And we aren't.*

We were taught that we needed to follow the myths and principles of EN in order to be loved and accepted. Remember, though, *that lesson is a lie.* In courageously speaking our truth, we follow Emerson's guidance and let go of the lies of EN.

# 7

# Victim Energy

"Never be bullied into silence. Never allow yourself
to be made a victim. Accept no one's definition
of your life; define yourself."

*Harvey Fierstein*

One common outcome of everyday narcissism is what I call *victim energy*.

First, let me make clear that victimization can be real. If you're walking down the street and are hit by lightning, or struck by a falling brick, or injured by a rock thrown by a mentally ill stranger, or shot by a police officer who fears that your cell phone is a gun—in that moment, you're genuinely a victim. However, it's important to see your victimization as a temporary state, not a way of life.

A victim is anyone who has been harmed, who has no other choices, and who is powerless to change his or her situation. For example, six-year-old Emilio is regularly beaten by his father. Emilio has no choice in what is happening to him and no power to stop the abuse. Each time he is beaten, he is a victim.

Now let's fast-forward a dozen years. Emilio is now eighteen, with normal intelligence and no disabilities, and he is larger than his dad. If his father tries to beat Emilio, he now *does* have some choices, although they're all painful. He can leave home. He can fight back. He can report the attempted abuse to the police or some other authority. He can tell his father, "If you try to hurt me, I'll punch your lights out *and* have you arrested." Or, he can wrestle his dad to the ground and tell him calmly, "You're never going to hurt me again. Ever. For any reason. I'll let you up when you say you understand and agree. Not before."

As many of us grew up and the myths and principles of EN were reinforced in us, over and over, by almost everyone we encountered, we were often powerless and victimized. We had no choice; we had to follow the rules, both the useful and the harmful ones; we had to live according to the principles and myths of EN. While we were growing up, all of this may have been true.

Now, though, as adults, we do not have to be bound by these myths and principles. Each of us has the freedom and the ability to grow out of them, to leave them by the side of the road as we journey forward.[3]

Leaving the myths and principles behind is of course somewhat easier said than done. If you were raised to please others and not take your own wants and needs seriously, then you may feel victimized by the people in your life who continue to tell you, "You're responsible for making me feel safe and happy."

As an adult, however, you *do* have choices. You can choose to set boundaries for yourself. You can choose to say no to other people's requests. You can pay attention to your own wants and needs, and to the promptings of your heart. And when someone says, "What's wrong with you? You're so selfish and inflexible!," you can say no once again, propose an alternative, or walk away. Each of these choices is healthy, empowering, and healing.

Our EN encourages us to do just the opposite—to think of ourselves as powerless victims and to see our victimhood as an ongoing state of being. This is rarely conscious. Few of us think or say, "I'm a victim. That's my lot in life." Yet, because of our EN, it's how many of us often act.

---

3    There are some genuine situations in which adults can be victimized. For example, having a serious disability or illness may reduce your power and limit your choices.

When we think of ourselves as victims, we don't have to take risks. We don't have to step into the uncertainty of life. We can simply stay stuck where we are, blame other people (or our situation, or our culture, or God), and try to get everyone else to change. We can stand in our EN and say to others, "*You're* the problem. *You're* the reason I'm stuck and victimized. *You* need to change. Change in exactly the way I want. Then, at last, you'll make me happy." This is a combination of Myth 2 and victim energy.

## Victim energy keeps us from taking positive action.

We declare ourselves as a victim whenever we whine, gossip, complain, or get angry—either aloud to others, or mentally to ourselves—without doing anything to improve our situation. We tell ourselves we're victims when things don't go exactly the way we want: when our car breaks down, when our cat vomits on the table, when our children fight, when our partner ignores us, or when our picnic gets rained out. Yet we know perfectly well that cars break, cats barf, kids fight, partners need time alone, and rain falls.

Victim energy keeps us from taking positive action. It keeps us in our anger and self-pity—and it keeps our heart closed. And, often, it keeps us from feeling—and dealing with—what is really bothering us. As we will see in a later chapter, victim energy can be one of the main ways in which we distract ourselves from feeling our own woundedness, grief, or loss.

Victim energy can be both subtle and insidious. If you say to your daughter in a whiny voice, "Jane, how many times do I have to tell you to hang up your coat?," that's a mild form of victim energy and EN. This is very different from, "Jane, I've asked you to hang up your coat three times. Now I'm turning off the TV until you do." It is said as a matter of fact, with no threats or whining.

The core message in these words isn't about your feelings, Jane's ostensible responsibility to take care of them, or her badness or wrongness. It's *You have certain responsibilities in our home, and there will be consequences if you don't fulfill them.* (It's also a very different message from "Hang up your coat *now* or you'll regret it." That is both threatening and potentially abusive.)

Whining in general is an expression of victim energy. When we whine *at* someone about something they said or did, we convey this core message: *You made me miserable. Your role is to make me happy, and you did the opposite. That makes you very bad.* Here we see Myths 2 and 5 in action.

It's also easy for us to write stories in our heads about the awful things that could happen—stories in which we will be victimized in some way. If we try to return a sweater that doesn't fit, we may imagine that the store clerk will belittle us, victimize us, and not let us return the sweater. If we ask our neighbor to turn down his stereo after 11:00 p.m., we might imagine that he'll become our lifelong enemy. If we purchase a sofa and the front leg falls off two days later, we may imagine that customer service will not help us with the repair. Yet these are all just fearful mental scenarios—stories we have written in our head, not accurate predictions. When they bubble up, as they naturally will, we can note them for what they are—stories of imaginary victimization—shrug them off, and get on with our life.

In one common variant of these mental scenarios, we imagine that if we do something differently, or less than perfectly, we will be victimized by someone's judgment, anger, or rejection. In another common variation, we imagine the calamities that might befall us if *someone else* fails to do everything perfectly. Behind all of these mental whirlpools is a sense that the world is waiting to victimize us.

## MARCIA

As Marcia drives to work one fall morning, she feels grateful for the beautiful day, the deep blue sky, the newly surfaced road, and the new car she is driving. She is looking forward to her workday. She is happy.

Then a thought about Christmas drops into her head. The holiday is almost three months away. She realizes that she will probably spend it by herself this year. Her daughter will be in California with her girlfriend, visiting her parents. Her brother will be busy with his large family. Her father, may he rest in peace, died the previous Christmas Eve. She misses him terribly. She fears that throughout the holidays she will be isolated and alone.

Marcia wipes a tear from her face. Soon she is weeping steadily.

Two miles later, with tears still flowing, Marcia realizes that *nothing has changed.* Nothing has happened except that she wrote a story in her head. She is still in same car, on the same road, on the same gorgeous fall morning, driving to the same job that she enjoys. Yet for the last two minutes she cried her eyes out.

However, she realizes her tears were victim tears. As Marcia drove, she wrote a mental story about being alone and lonely on Christmas. She started feeling sorry for herself that her daughter wouldn't want to spend Christmas with her. Then she realized her misery was all over events that literally had not happened—and perhaps never would.

Marcia laughs. She comes back to the present and resumes enjoying her drive.

Eleven weeks later, Marcia does spend Christmas alone, with a fire in her fireplace and one of her favorite meals. She finds it very relaxing and cozy. To her surprise, she enjoys not being caught up in the Christmas frazzle and hustle. She decides she wants more Christmases like this one in the future.

---

Usually when we fall into victim energy, we aren't actually victims at all. We just think of ourselves that way. Ninety percent of the time, we have choices—sometimes plenty of them—even when we think, or imagine, that we don't. The choices may be difficult, or painful, or unpleasant, or frightening; yet they are still choices. Nevertheless, we tell ourselves that we are victims because none of the choices satisfy us, and all of them are scary, uncomfortable, or painful to execute.

Furthermore, often when we think we haven't made a choice, we have—even when we thought we had no choices. If you live in a small town with only one public high school, you may imagine that you have no choice; you have to send your teenage daughter there. Yet you *do* have choices. You can homeschool her. You can hire a tutor to give her additional instruction in the evenings or on weekends. You can move to a different school district. You can organize a group of local parents to establish a small charter school. You can pay to send her to the Catholic school forty miles away and drive her to and from school each day (or get her a car so she can drive herself).

I'm not saying any of these options is easy, or necessarily better. I'm simply observing that if you say to yourself, *I guess we just have to send her to the local high school,* you're putting a victim's spin on the situation. You actually *have* made a choice. Think how much more positive and empowering this thought would be: *We've considered all the options and decided on the local high school; it's not ideal, and we wish we had better alternatives. Given the circumstances, though, we believe it's the best way to go.*

One easy way to tell if you are stuck in victim energy is if you whine or complain—either aloud to others, or silently to yourself—for more than a few moments. Another sign of victim energy is when you think that you are powerless and stuck, that you have no choices. And when you stay angry, rather than feel a brief flash of anger and then let it go, you are very likely acting from Myth 2 and victim energy.

Yet victim energy is itself a choice. We choose the pain of seeing ourselves as a victim because it's easier than being responsible. We choose victim energy because it's easier to blame someone else—or events, or our culture, or God—than to take responsibility for our own well-being.

Being responsible doesn't mean expecting ourselves to be able to control the outcome of our choices. Life is always uncertain. Sometimes when we make a choice, we get the results we expected or hoped for. Sometimes, because of events beyond our influence, the results are wildly different, or even the opposite or what we wanted. However, this doesn't make us a victim. It makes us human. It also gives us the opportunity to learn from what happened and make another choice—and then another and another and another, as life continually unfolds.

Our EN tells us that we have to make the perfect choice every time, and if we don't, it's because we are bad or defective or shameful. This is yet another lie, because *every time we make our best choice, we are caring for ourselves, no matter what the eventual outcome is.*

## SHELLY

Shelly has worked for a large corporation for many years and, until recently, has been reasonably happy there. A few months ago, however, a series of austerity measures changed everything. Suddenly she and her coworkers were asked to do much more with fewer people. Her boss told her, "You don't have to work harder—just smarter." Shelley and her boss both knew this was nonsense.

Shelly's company is in a service industry. Because of the cutbacks, many clients have received poor services. They naturally complained, and morale at work suffered.

Each day over lunch, Shelly and her coworkers commiserate about the situation. After lunch, she returns to work thinking of herself, her colleagues, and her clients as victims.

After a few months, however, Shelly has had enough of victim energy. She is done with feeling distraught and tired every afternoon. She realizes that she has the power to choose.

First, she chooses not to go to those lunches any more. They sap her energy and make her afternoons very long.

Second, she realizes that she always has the choice to leave her job and look for a better one. However, for now, she decides to stay because she likes the salary, the working hours, and the benefits.

Third, she chooses not to whine and complain anymore because she realizes that she has made the choice to stay and knows that she can always choose to leave.

When Shelly steps out of victim energy, something unexpected happens: her anger dissipates and her heart opens. Now she knows fully what she has been feeling. What bubbles up—and what she courageously steps into—are sadness, discouragement, and disappointment.

As Shelly lets herself feel these emotions in the weeks that follow, she realizes that she does need to leave the organization. However, she is doing this as her choice—because she wants something better—not because she's a victim. She is choosing to leave for her own serenity and happiness.

Shelly gives notice and leaves, feeling relieved and powerful. A few weeks later she begins a new and much more rewarding career, with a more open and hopeful heart.

Because of our EN, it's easy for any of us, even therapists, to fall into victim energy sometimes. The good news is that simply noticing you're in victim energy is the first and most important step of breaking free from it. In fact, you may be surprised at how easy it may sometimes be to reorient yourself once you recognize that you're thinking like a victim.

This is no panacea or magic bullet, however. Some of us have been more deeply traumatized than others—and the deeper your trauma, the more work it may take for you to be able to repeatedly make this turn. For example, if you were deeply traumatized in childhood by physical abuse or incest, you will likely need a lot of time and practice to develop the habit of recognizing and releasing victim energy. Nevertheless, it is a practice you can learn, and one that other people with similar experiences have learned as well.

---

## HEALING ACTIVITY #11

### Step Out of Victim Energy

Here's an easy-to-follow overview of what to look for —and what to do—to free yourself from victim energy.

| If you find yourself... | Here is how to quickly break out of victim energy. |
|---|---|
| Whining to others | Speak more firmly and in a lower register. Use short, straightforward sentences. At the end of each sentence, lower the pitch of your voice, so that people hear a period instead of a question mark or exclamation point. Use the same tone of voice you would in a job interview. Straighten your back so you stand or sit up straight. |
| Complaining to others | Simply stop. If you feel you absolutely must complain, give yourself exactly thirty seconds. Time yourself as you complain. At the end of thirty seconds, say aloud, "Done!" Then change the subject. |
| Gossiping | If you're the one gossiping about someone, stop and change the subject. If someone else is gossiping to you, change the subject, end the conversation, or excuse yourself and leave the room. |
| Whining or complaining to yourself | Name what you're doing. Say aloud, "I'm whining" or "Looks like I'm complaining." Then say, "I'm not a victim. I have choices." Take responsibility for the choices you have made so far regarding your situation; if you've blamed others for the situation, stop. Then move into practical action. Ask yourself, *What are my options?* Get a pen and a piece of paper, or open a computer file. Think about and create a numbered list with all the options you can think of for handling the situation. (Be sure to include as an option, *Accept the situation as it is, without trying to change it—and stop complaining about it.* This might—though it probably won't—be the choice you finally make. Do be sure to write this down, so you realize that it is a choice, not something you're stuck with.) |

| If you find yourself . . . | Here is how to quickly break out of victim energy. |
|---|---|
| All of the above | Remind yourself that you have choices; therefore, you are not a victim. Then do something about the situation. List all the options you can think of for improving things. Pick the option that seems most promising, and try it. If it works, keep doing it. If it doesn't, try something else. |

## SUE AND PHILANDRO

Sue has been a full-time homemaker for almost fifteen years. She and her husband, Philandro, have four children, ranging in age from five to fourteen.

Philandro lost his construction job two years ago, and he hasn't yet taken a new one. He has been offered several jobs in retail and manufacturing. The problem is that they've all paid less than half of what he made in construction, so he has turned them all down.

Although Sue understands why Philandro has said no to those jobs, she is somewhat angry and bitter that her husband hasn't been more diligent in his job search. She wishes he would be willing to settle for a much smaller salary rather than use most of their savings to keep the family afloat. As Sue watches their savings dwindle, she feels stuck and victimized. Philandro has been the family's sole breadwinner for many years, and Sue feels powerless to alter their financial situation. She has told Philandro many times how afraid she is of running out of money. Each time, though, he just nods and says, "I know, hon; I'm doing my best" or "Don't worry about the money, baby; we're okay."

One day after working on releasing her EN and victim energy, Sue realizes she isn't actually powerless at all. She announces to Philandro, "I'm going to get a full-time job. I'm not willing for us to go broke while you keep job hunting and holding out for a higher salary. And if we both end up working, that's good, too. After a few years, we can replenish our savings and be back to where we were before you got laid off." Then she adds, "In the meantime, until you're back to work, I want you to spend more time with the kids and take on more of your responsibility around the house."

At first Philandro gets angry and tells her it's not necessary for her to work. She starts applying for jobs anyway.

Two months later, Sue gets a full-time job in a bookstore. Although Sue is somewhat bitter about having to go to work for a small salary, she feels some relief that she is slowing the depletion of her family's savings. She is able to relax somewhat about money.

Three months after that, Philandro finds a new construction job, and a week later they are both working full-time. Soon they are financially stable once again and able to resume putting money aside each month.

Instead of listening to her own victim energy, Sue listened to the needs that were speaking to her: her need for financial security and her need for self-respect. Instead of continuing to try to get her husband to empathize with her fear and bring in a steady income, she took action herself. Because of her decision to go back to work, she felt more empowered, less fearful, and more cared for.

Soon another problem appears, however. For almost fifteen years, Sue has been responsible for all the household duties and care of the children. Now she simply doesn't have the time. Most days, when she comes home after a long day at work, the kitchen is a mess. Philandro, who gets home two hours before she does, usually cooks dinner. Sue appreciates this, especially since her husband is a talented cook. However, Philandro rarely cleans up afterward, and he's sloppy.

Sue explains to her husband how important it is for her to come home to a reasonably clean kitchen. He nods and promises to do better. Yet, as Sue eventually learns, having a clean kitchen simply isn't important to Philandro.

Sue finds herself becoming angrier and more bitter every time she returns home to a messy kitchen. She feels like a victim of her husband's lack of concern and his unwillingness to change to meet her needs.

Then Sue decides to once again listen to her own feelings and needs. She tells her husband, "I'm tired of nagging you about the kitchen, and I know you're sick of it, too. I'm going to hire one of the neighborhood teenagers to come over on weekday evenings to clean the kitchen. They can clean while we eat." Philandro kisses her on the forehead and says, "Great idea."

By listening to her feelings and needs and trusting them, Sue was able to create a solution to meet those needs. As it turned out, her husband appreciated each solution as well.

Sue and Philandro still don't have a perfect marriage. Nevertheless, Sue feels much happier on a day-to-day basis.

# Shame: The Outcome of Everyday Narcissism

"Every child, every person needs to know
that they are a source of joy ... "

*Jean Vanier*

When we're told over and over that who we are is not okay, that rules are more important than we are, and that other people matter and we don't, we do more than just shut down our true selves. We also develop shame.

When we're in shame, we feel exposed, vulnerable, and worthless, all at once. It is the most painful emotion we can experience. Yet, unlike anger, fear, or disappointment, shame is not innate to the human organism. It is learned.

Shame is also a cycle, a downward spiral. Over time, it causes us to hide our true self deeper and deeper, so others can't see how worthless we feel we truly are.

After years of hiding our perceived worthlessness from others, we eventually hide it from ourselves as well—behind defenses such as anger, blame, rationalizing, intellectualizing, addictions, self-pity, self-righteousness, analyzing, defiance, perfectionism, or any of a hundred others. These defenses block our healing and keep us from feeling our shame.

> ... not feeling our shame prevents us from healing it.

Much of our shame comes from our secrets—the things we've decided no one can know about us because they would surely judge us and reject us if they knew. Secrets are like cancer to our self-esteem. The longer we keep them to ourselves, the more damage they do. They eat away at us.

Over time, we can get so proficient at hiding behind our defenses that we don't even consciously feel our shame when it arises. Sadly, not feeling our shame prevents us from healing it. The impact of all this is profoundly negative. It reduces our ability to be honest with ourselves and others and it impairs our ability to have happy, fulfilling relationships.

Like EN itself, and most other EN wounds, we begin developing shame before we turn five. Its development continues throughout our childhood and adolescence and gets perpetuated in adulthood. It is then passed on from one generation to the next—to our own children, to their children, and beyond.

### *Should* and Shame

We commonly use the word *should* in a variety of ways:

- Adults often use *should* to teach children what, in adults' opinion, is the right thing to do or not do. *(You should always say "please" and "thank you.")*

- All of us use *should* when giving advice to others. *(You should never trust a car salesman.)*

- Many of us use *should* to manipulate others by shaming them. *(If you want to be a good grandchild, you should buy your granddad a birthday gift.)*

Most of us use the world *should* regularly, without thinking. However, the word is often a form of coercion. Much of the time we use it to define for others—and, often, for ourselves—what is right or good. If we accept and obey the *should*, then we are good people; if we don't, we are bad. Since none of us wants to see ourselves—or be seen by others—as bad, we feel forced to obey each *should*.

Thus, in our hunger to belong and be loved, we learn to follow many of the *shoulds* taught to us through Myth 5: *we are not lovable as we are; we can only become lovable through what we do and say.* The *shoulds* tell us what we need to do or say to belong and make ourselves lovable. Because of our EN, we believe that if we consistently do all of those *shoulds*, then we will be loved or cared for.

It's not just the word *should* that's so toxic. It's also the concept behind it, whether or not the word is explicitly used.

In all kinds of relationships, most of us use *should* to shame other people into doing things that conflict with their own truths. Worse yet, most of us also use it to shame *ourselves* into doing things that conflict with *our* own truths. And all the while, we are unaware of what we are doing—and of the wounding this creates. By the time most of us reach adulthood, *should* has become a staple of our thinking and being.

## ISABEL AND SAM

Sam, Isabel's five-year-old son, comes running into the room, slamming the door behind him. He's excited to show his mother a picture he made of a bunny, with cotton for the tail and felt for the ears. He is very proud. He yells, "Mom!"

Isabel doesn't respond right away because she's on the phone, making a doctor appointment for her elderly mother. In fact, she turns away from her son so she can better hear the receptionist on the other end of the line.

To get her attention, Sam yells "MOM!" a couple of more times. This makes Isabel's phone conversation impossible. She finally shouts in an angry and disgusted tone, "Not now, Sam!"

Sam starts to cry. He is confused about what he did wrong to get his mother to react in such a way. Mentally, he runs off a list of *shoulds* he has learned: *you shouldn't let the door slam; you shouldn't shout at someone who's in the same room; you shouldn't talk to Mom when she is on the phone.*

Because of Sam's EN, he comes to the conclusion that his mom's anger is all his fault. Although he is far too young to even know what a myth is, he is already practicing Myths 1, 3, 4, and 5. He thinks that if only he'd come into the room the right way, by following all the rules he'd learned, she'd have swept him into her arms, kissed him on the cheek, and said, "Let me see that bunny!"

Sam is young and his world is small. In his mind, whatever happens in the world is because of him. He doesn't understand that Isabel was happy to see him and simply needed to complete her phone call before turning her attention to him. So he decides that he didn't get the love he wanted because he didn't do what he *should* have. He didn't follow all the rules, so he had to pay the price of his mother's anger and rejection—which he believes are his fault.

---

As children, we are told over and over that we *should* finish our homework, do our chores, pick up our room, go to a family event, wear our hair differently, and so on. Eventually we internalize the message that if we want to be loved and accepted, we need to give up our choices and do what we *should*. Almost always, this means doing what others want and not respecting our own desires and needs.

As we grow older, we gather more and more *shoulds* that we are taught we need to follow. Now, as adults, the word *should* haunts most of us because of our EN. We continue to allow it to coerce us to do things in order to belong. In short, the word *should* falsely assures us that we are indeed good and worthy of love—*if* we do what we're told we *should*.

When we hear the word, even in our own thoughts, we respond from the terrified child within us. We feel this response in our body. That child believes (or fears) that we did something wrong—rather than what we should have—and is desperate to learn and follow all the *shoulds* in order to belong and be loved.

This is how some of us develop severe anxiety or guilt over the possibility that we didn't do or say the right thing—or might fail to do or say it in the future. Our adult heads are full of innumerable *shoulds* to draw upon. When something goes wrong, we fall into Myth 1, rapidly go through this list of *shoulds*, and come up with three or four things that we should have done differently to make the person happy. If only we had done things *that* way, our EN tells us, we would have gotten exactly the love, acceptance, and other things we wanted.

These *shoulds* control much of our lives. Sometimes they turn a simple statement or task into a source of enormous anxiety and guilt. For example, we say to ourselves, *I should do the dishes now. If I do them now, it means I'm a good mother and wife and human being, and that I'm responsible, clean, and organized. However, if I don't wash the dishes now, as I've been told I should, then I'm a bad wife and mother and person; I'm irresponsible, lazy, dirty, and disorganized.*

Thus, we coerce ourselves into acting in certain ways—and, in the process, wound ourselves yet again.

At the heart of the self-coercion is the desire to not be a bad human being. Of course, not doing the dishes wouldn't make anyone a bad person. There are plenty of honorable reasons to choose not to do the dishes. We might be tired or sick. Or we might prefer to play with our children before they go to bed. (Washing the dishes doesn't make anyone a better or more likable person, either. We can wash dishes all day and still have others say that we're very difficult to be around.) Washing the dishes right now is a choice, yet we present it to ourselves as a moral necessity.

Our EN turns everyday choices into value judgments. It tells us that, depending on what choice we make, we are either likable or unlikable, either lovable or unlovable, either good or bad. However, choosing to wash or not wash the dishes right now has *nothing* to do with our value as a human being. We all have value, no matter what we do (or don't do) with our dirty dishes, or anything else.

Value judgments are qualitatively different from discernment. *Discernment* is the ability to recognize a situation for what it is and make mindful choices based on that reality. *Judgment* operates in a completely different way, by labeling a person as good or bad, right or wrong, lovable or unlovable.

To heal from our EN, we need to learn to let go of our collection of *shoulds*, as well as our value judgments about ourselves. We need to be gentle with ourselves. We need to forgive ourselves for our humanness. As we learn to do this, we also become less judgmental of others.

Releasing our *shoulds* and judgments in turn releases our anxiety, shame, and guilt. As these fall away, we discover more opportunities for loving ourselves.

## Moving beyond Shame

The good news is that, because shame is learned, it can also be unlearned. The activity that follows will help you steadily unlearn your shame day by day, through one encounter after another.

---

## HEALING ACTIVITY #12

---

### Notice and Let Go of Shame

Here are some ways to begin recognizing, naming, and healing from shame:

- Notice how often you use the word *should* in talking with others. For the first three to four days, actually count the number of times you hear yourself say it each day. (Note: the *actual* number will likely be four to five times the number you notice and tally up.)

- Notice how often—with others and with yourself—you *think* the word *should*.

- Notice how often you hear others use the word *should*.

- Pay attention to how your body feels when you speak or think the word.

- Pay attention to how your body feels when *someone else* uses it in talking to you.

- As much as possible, avoid using the word *should*—in what you say, what you write, and even what you think. Instead, replace the word with specific consequences. For example, if you notice yourself thinking, *I should wash the dishes now*, stop for a moment. Then think through the *realistic* consequences of doing versus not doing the dishes right now. For example: *If I do the dishes tonight, I'll feel good making breakfast in a clean kitchen tomorrow morning. On the other hand, I'm really tired; if I go to bed early and do the dishes in the morning, I'll be able to get almost an hour of extra sleep.* Be sure to notice that neither choice has anything to do with being a good, decent, lovable human being; instead, each choice presents its own set of likely consequences.

- When others impose the word *should* on you, ignore its shaming and EN overtones. Instead, mentally replace the word with specific consequences, as you learned to do when the word appeared in your own thoughts.

## Defenses

Because shame can be so painful, we develop internal defenses that protect us from feeling it fully—or at all. These defenses arise from a desperate need to make sure that people don't see how flawed we are (or, more accurately, how flawed we *think* we are). Without even being aware of it, we believe that if others saw our flaws, they would judge us, find us wanting, reject us, and, of course, not love us.

Shame is especially easy for someone else to trigger in us—sometimes with nothing more than a disgusted look, a terse comment, a criticism, or an angry tone of voice. And when an event triggers our shame, the shame in turn instantly triggers our defenses. We rush in with these defenses to prove to others (and ourselves) that they are seeing us incorrectly; that the flaws they observe aren't real; that we are not the bad person they think we are—the person our EN has taught *us* to believe we are.

> Shame is especially easy for someone else to trigger in us—sometimes with nothing more than a disgusted look, a terse comment, a criticism, or an angry tone of voice.

Over time, these defenses become so habitual that we no longer feel much of our shame. Our defenses thus keep us from feeling worthless, unlovable, or exposed. They help us avoid wishing we could disappear. In that sense, they protect us from some emotional pain. However, these defenses also prevent us from knowing what is really going on inside us. They protect us from our own true feelings. This makes us less able to know and care for ourselves.

Like an infected physical wound, unhealed shame stays in our body indefinitely. Although our defenses temporarily protect us from some of the pain of shame, they also keep it from healing.

The list of common defenses is quite long. It includes blame, fury, self-pity, self-righteousness, addictions, gossiping, intellectualizing, overanalyzing, running away (physically or emotionally), bullying, defiance, perfectionism, anger, virtuosity, and several dozen others. These defenses all block our healing.

## HEALING ACTIVITY #13

### Recognize Your Defenses and Heal Your Shame

Here are some practices to help you become more aware of your own defenses, so you can let them dissolve and then heal the shame behind them:

- Make a conscious commitment to feel your shame, and accept the pain of it, rather than defend yourself against it.

- Ask yourself what defenses you typically use to avoid feeling shame. Reflect on this question. Then in your healing notebook, or in a computer file, create a list of all the defenses you recognize. Common defenses include anger, blame, confusion, self-righteousness, self-pity, rationalizing, analyzing, intellectualizing, denial, victim energy, and addictive behavior.

- Think back and reflect on some situations in which you used your defenses to protect yourself from others' potentially painful judgments. What forms did those defenses take? If any of these are not already on your list of defenses, add them.

- In the weeks and months to come, as you recall other past events and live into current ones, note any other defenses that you observe. Add these to your list.

- Review your list of defenses at least once a day. As you familiarize yourself with this list, you will gradually become aware of which ones you tend to choose.

The next steps are painful, yet deeply valuable:

- From now on, whenever you notice one of your defenses arising, don't throw yourself into it. Instead, choose to *not* use it—or, if you've already begun to use it, drop it, and step back from it.

- Then let yourself feel the shame that sits just behind that defense. Counterintuitive as this sounds, allowing yourself to feel this shame is the key to healing from it, growing beyond it, and letting it fall away. It doesn't matter whether you're with someone or alone; whether someone is watching you or not; or whether someone knows (or seems to know) what you're thinking or feeling. Simply let the shame arise. For a few moments, feel it and let it be, without doing anything to it or about it. Let yourself feel bad, unworthy, or unlovable.

- Then, test the validity of that feeling by finding out if the people around you feel the same way about you. Say to them, "Please help me with something. I just said or did _____, and now I'm feeling shameful because of it. I'd like to ask you three questions:

  - "Based on what I said or did (e.g., I interrupted you, got angry, sounded stupid, or raised my voice), do you think less of me?"

  - "Do you still like (or love) me?"

  - "Do *you* think I'm bad?"

These questions sound childlike because they are. When you feel shame, you are in a childlike state. The child inside you is hungry to know that you are not bad, that you are indeed lovable or likable.

Because of your and others' EN, you were not allowed to ask these questions when you were a child. Now, however, as an adult, you can honor yourself—and give that part of yourself a voice—by asking these questions.

Your healing actually begins as you listen to your shame and ask the questions. Over time, as you continue to ask the questions, you'll discover that the way others answer the questions doesn't matter as much as loving yourself enough to ask them.

The adult part of your psyche knows that most people will give positive answers to these questions, most of the time. The child inside you doesn't know this, though. That child needs to be given permission by your inner adult to ask these questions.

When you do begin asking others these questions, it's important to ask them only of people you trust—people you know will be both honest and compassionate. They will tell the truth in a way that is empowering, not demeaning, even if their truth may hurt initially.

As difficult as these questions are to ask at first, the process will get easier and easier with practice. Over time, you will build a positive and empowering habit. The more you ask these questions of others when shame appears, the more your shame will heal, and the more your fear and anxiety will dissipate. The myths and principles of EN will look and feel ever more hollow, and eventually they will fade away entirely.

Shame is like the grass clippings left over from mowing your lawn. If you put the clippings in a bag and seal it, the grass will start to decompose. If you ignore the bag long enough, it may even spontaneously combust. That's just what shame does when we keep our shame-wrapped secrets inside us. It eats away at our self-esteem and self-confidence.

However, if we open the bag of grass clippings and spread them on our garden, some of them will dry up and blow away; the rest will become beneficial fertilizer. Shame works the same way. Once we open up to others and expose our shame and secrets to the air, we discover that people don't think less of us. They still like us and don't think we are bad. Then healing can begin, and shame can be replaced with comfort and love.

> Once we open up to others and expose our shame and secrets to the air, we discover that people don't think less of us.

Eventually you will want to ask the three clarifying questions because you will have discovered how much better you feel after you give voice to them. You will also discover that most other people do not judge you as harshly as you learned to judge yourself years ago. In fact, you'll discover that many people will respond to your childlike questions with comments such as "I think more of you now because of the courage it took to ask the questions," or "I like you even more now because I know you better and respect the journey you are on."

None of us heals in isolation. Relationships are our container for healing. We need other people's perspectives on us because ours has been distorted through our EN. We also need to share our feelings with others. And as we do, we discover that others rarely think as badly about us as we think about ourselves.

I've been a therapist for over thirty years. In all this time, only once have I heard someone answer the three questions with, "Yeah, I do think less of you." And that was from someone who was harsh and judgmental about *everyone,* including herself. Otherwise, people have been supportive and kind.

---

## HEALING ACTIVITY #14

### Love the Child inside You

Here's one more activity to practice regularly that will allow you to love yourself more deeply:

- Find three or four photographs of yourself when you were very young. Frame each one nicely. Display them in highly visible spots around your home. If possible, display one at work as well.

- Several times a day, look at one or more of these photos. Notice your preciousness when you were small. Recognize the deep desire in that young person to be adored, liked, and loved. Remember how vulnerable you were then. Send that small human being—your younger self—some loving, healing energy.

- Then acknowledge how vulnerable part of you still is. Promise yourself that when someone is being hard on you, or when you are being hard on yourself, you will remember that precious child within. This child is trying hard to be a decent human being, to be kind and compassionate and wise.

- When you get upset with yourself, whether for something in the present or something in the past, remember that you are being hard on this small, vulnerable person within you. Stop judging that little human being; bless them instead. Tell yourself that your intentions are and were honorable, even if you don't always succeed. Also tell yourself that you will love the little child within, no matter what anybody else does. Remind yourself of just how precious you were—and are.

- Explain to yourself that, as a child, you really did nothing wrong. You were just a small, young person trying to figure out the world. All the rejection and anger and disgust and dismissiveness you experienced from others was not your fault.

- Reassure your younger self that they no longer need to follow the myths or principles of EN—and that you love them just as they are. Explain to them that they are a good person at heart, even though they don't always express that goodness. They will sometimes make mistakes; however, that is part of being human. Tell your younger self that you will not criticize them for mistakes, and that you are learning new skills to take care of them.

- Please repeat this activity regularly, day after day and week after week. As you do, you will love yourself more deeply. Your heart will steadily open, and, day by day, your EN will heal.

The activities in this chapter are difficult and, at first, painful to practice. Yet they are healing on many levels. As you practice, you will also discover something paradoxical about your emotions: they are sometimes very simple and childlike. Yet all your healing, solutions, and growth will come from you as an adult.

# Distracting Ourselves
# and Each Other

"People will seek the ends of the galaxy to avoid
that which they need most."

*Criss Jami*

As you have begun to discover, the only genuine cure for emotional pain begins with accepting it, feeling it fully, addressing it, and moving through it. This heals the wound behind the pain. Paradoxically, accepting and feeling emotional pain is the key to putting an end to that pain.

> . . . the only genuine cure for emotional pain
> begins with accepting it, feeling it fully,
> addressing it, and moving through it.

In practice, however, most of us try to avoid our emotional pain rather than heal it. Instead of healing our emotional wounds, we try to distract ourselves from our pain. Partly this is because, as kids, we were never given permission to feel or taught how to deal with our emotions. Partly it's because we have such a wide variety of readily available options for distracting ourselves.

We distract ourselves in hundreds of different ways, with hundreds of different thoughts, activities, or obsessions. These distractions help us go numb. Going numb closes our heart and disconnects us from ourselves and our bodies. This prevents our heart from healing.

When unpleasant feelings begin to arise in us, we may turn to our distractors to avoid experiencing those feelings. This avoidance can occur so rapidly and so automatically that we often aren't aware of it. To heal your EN, you need to notice this reflexive habit and change it.

Most distractors are activities. Some are thoughts we compulsively or habitually dwell on. And some distractors are other emotions: we distract ourselves from what we don't want to feel by feeling a different emotion instead. We numb ourselves to one feeling by throwing ourselves into another.

> When unpleasant feelings begin to arise in us, we may turn to our distractors to avoid experiencing those feelings.

Often we do this with shame, which is one of the most painful emotions. In order to avoid feeling exposed, worthless, and vulnerable, all at the same time, we may turn to anger, self-righteousness, or self-pity.

Each of us has our own favorite distractors. A full list of distractors would fill a small book. I'll spare you that book-length list. However, here are the most common ones.

## COMMON DISTRACTORS

Alcohol

Analyzing

Anger

Arrogance

Blame

Blogging

Children (caring for them, thinking about them, etc.)

Chores

Cleaning

Clubbing

Computer games

Complaining

Dating

Defiance

Denial

Drugs

Eating

Email

Entertaining (planning and hosting social events, etc.)

Exercising

Facebook

Fantasizing

Fear

Food (cooking, collecting recipes, planning menus, etc.)

Gambling

Gardening

Googling

Gossiping

Hand work (crocheting, needlepoint, embroidery, etc.)

Hobbies

Home maintenance and repair

Hosting or organizing events

Humor

Intellectualizing

Knitting

Judging others

Lying (either to others or to ourselves)

Meditation

Minimizing

Organizing (our home, our possessions, etc.)

Phoning

Playing sports

Pleasing others

Politics

Prayer

Pouting

Quilting

Rationalizing

Reading

Relationships

Religion

Revenge

Romance

School

Scrapbooking

Sex (having it, thinking about it, and fantasizing about it)

Shopping

Smoking or other tobacco use

Social media

Socializing

Television

Texting

Twitter

Victim energy

Volunteering

Video games

Videos and movies

Watching sports

Weight loss or management

Work

Writing mental stories

Yard work

As you can see, some normally virtuous activities—meditation, relationships, prayer, cleaning, volunteer work, etc.—can be used as distractors. That doesn't mean they aren't worthwhile or that it's best to not do them at all; just don't use them as a way to avoid feeling your emotional pain.

## PEMA CHÖDRÖN

In her audio presentation *Getting Unstuck*, Buddhist teacher Pema Chödrön tells the story of being at a retreat with several friends. At dinner, as they gathered, one of her friends refused to look at her, talk to her, or acknowledge her in any way. Because of her own everyday narcissism, most notably Myth 1, Chödrön felt very uneasy about this. She assumed her friend was behaving that way because of something Chödrön had said or done.

After dinner, Chödrön went to her room and meditated for an hour, hoping to alleviate her uneasiness. If you have meditated, you know how blissful it can feel. There is often peace, contentment, and a knowing that however things go, all will be well.

This was true for Chödrön. After her meditation, she was no longer bothered by her friend. Her uneasiness was gone. Yet Chödrön had mostly used meditation to try to distract herself from that uneasiness. So, as the hours passed, the uneasy feeling surfaced again.

At 1:00 in the morning, she got out of bed, unable to sleep. Continuing to feel uneasy, she went to the chapel to simply sit with her uneasiness instead of distracting herself with meditation. Soon she started sobbing. Her heart opened. She cried hard for about an hour.

During that process she got in touch with how she had spent her entire life trying to please others. Her meditation had actually distracted her from knowing what was in her heart.

This was a painful and wonderful awakening for Chödrön. She realized how hard she had tried to be liked and to belong. In doing so, she hadn't valued herself.

Now her healing could begin. She could take care of that wound.

---

## SARAH

A few years ago, I was in a group of women who gathered to explore and share their spiritual journeys. The women were asked to think about what they used to avoid their feelings— in other words, what distractors they typically employed.

Sarah spoke up with a surprised look on her face. She had suddenly realized how being extremely responsible— something she was regularly praised for and had always considered virtuous—was her primary distractor.

She was a dedicated teacher, mother, neighbor, church member, friend, homemaker, gardener, daughter, and sister. She frequently received accolades for how hard she worked. However, she now realized how these responsibilities left her with no quiet time for herself, no time to be with her own heart. This virtue kept her heart closed, kept her unaware of how she was feeling.

She realized she had used this distractor to avoid difficulties with her husband and her father. By keeping busy, she was consistently responsible to others—and not to herself.

---

## HEALING ACTIVITY #15

### Name Your Distractors

Now I'd like you to spend a few minutes identifying your own preferred distractors.

Review the list of distractors near the beginning of this chapter (and again near the end of this book). As you do, create a list of all of the distractors you use. Put this list in your healing notebook.

Remember, this isn't a list of what you *do*. Most of us routinely do many of the things on the list. *It's about what you do to distract yourself from emotional pain.* If you're not sure whether to check a particular item, simply ask yourself, *Is this something I do when I'm feeling down and want to feel better?*

At the bottom of the list, please add any other distractors that come to mind and don't appear in the list provided in this book.

Next, review your own completed list from top to bottom once again. Circle the five distractors you use most frequently.

In the weeks and months ahead, whenever you get the urge to do one of these five activities, stop and ask yourself the following question: *Is there a feeling I'm trying to avoid? What might it be? What am I afraid of feeling?* If you like, go to the list of feelings in this book for assistance. Remember that the answers to these questions may involve multiple emotions.

If, in response to this question, an emotion starts to bubble up, find a place where you can sit down comfortably and quietly for a few minutes, alone. Then let those feelings rise up inside you. Instead of trying to wrestle with them or push them away, just let them be.

Then look at how you can begin taking care of yourself around those feelings. If you feel lonely, call a friend. If you feel confined, take a walk. If you feel powerless, do something that enables you to make a difference, such as volunteering for an organization you believe in, or cooking dinner for a sick friend.

Sometimes taking care of yourself doesn't mean doing anything more than examining your feelings with curiosity instead of fear for a few minutes, calmly letting them grow and then subside.

*Important:* if a distractor is helpful—e.g., meditation, work, cooking, gardening, volunteering—I am *not* asking you to stop doing it. Continue to make it a part of your life.

However, whenever you do engage in that activity, be aware of your motivations. Are you doing it because it brings you happiness or in some way helps other human beings? Or are you doing it to distract yourself from something you don't want to face? Are you engaging with life or trying to avoid it?

I also suggest you let go of any inherently unhelpful distractors, such as blaming, complaining, and revenge.

## Our Four Biggest Distractors

Although we can distract ourselves from most of our feelings in hundreds of different ways, in practice, we tend to rely on four major distractors:

- Anger
- Fear
- Attempting to please other people
- Victim energy

### ANGER

As children, most of us were not allowed to express—or even feel—much anger. Our anger obviously upset the adults around us. They firmly believed in Myth 2, so they let us know that their anger was fine, while ours would not be tolerated. As a result, most of us were never taught how to express our anger appropriately or how to use it effectively.

Yet we need our anger. It can be a great motivator. It informs us that something is wrong. And often it points to another emotion that resides underneath.

We usually get angry when we have been hurt, embarrassed, demeaned, discounted, or betrayed. However, our anger can easily distract us from this other, deeper pain. We may then choose to stay in our anger instead of exploring what is beneath it.

In some ways, this anger may actually feel good. We don't just get to avoid the pain underneath; we also get to feel more powerful and in control. It pushes many people away so we feel safer. Yet when we stay in our anger, our heart stays closed, and we may lash out and hurt others.

### PETER

When Peter first came to see me, he felt very depressed and confused. He and his wife, Samantha, had been having problems for several years. For the past year, he had paid for an apartment for her because she had told him she needed her own space.

Eventually Samantha told Peter she wanted a divorce. At the same time, she revealed that she had a boyfriend, and that he had been living with her in the apartment.

A few weeks after this discussion, Peter made an appointment with me.

Peter had learned long ago, early in life, to shut down his heart. He did this so thoroughly that, even in this situation, he could not feel any anger—only confusion and depression.

It took Peter a year of therapy to open his heart enough to begin to feel and express his anger. When he did, however, it took him only a few weeks to move past that anger into the emotions underneath it: shock, confusion, and betrayal. As he experienced, expressed, and moved through these feelings, his heart slowly came back to life.

## JOHN

John came to see me in therapy, hoping to save his marriage with Lucy. I quickly learned that John had a serious anger problem. He had hit Lucy with his fist during an argument. A court had granted her an order of protection.

In our second session, John explained that he had been regularly beaten as a child, as had all his siblings. In his family, the regular expression of anger by the adults—including throwing objects, knocking him on the back of his head, and slamming him against the wall—was considered normal.

I soon learned that John survived his childhood by shutting down his feelings, going numb, and closing his heart. It was the only way he could shield himself from an environment of constant fear, pain, and anger.

Eventually, numbness and anger became John's way of life and parts of his personality. Now they threatened his marriage.

It took well over a year—yet slowly, John began to open his heart. He started to feel his way beneath his anger, which had distracted him from his real issues. His healing had begun.

One by one, John was able to name these feelings: self-loathing, fear, powerlessness, and hopelessness. Over time, as he shared these feelings, he learned how to take care of them himself rather than expect Lucy to handle them for him. Week by week, he grew beyond the confines of Myth 2.

........................................................................................................

How we express our anger toward someone else says far more about us than about the person we are angry with.

For example, if we have learned that it is okay to combine our expression of anger with cruelty, criticism, or blame, then we'll say to someone who inadvertently bumped into us, "Hey, knucklehead! Are you always this clumsy, or are you just drunk?" And if we're angry with someone who arrived late, we'll say, "What's wrong with you? Dinner has been waiting for forty-five minutes!"

> How we express our anger toward someone
> else says far more about us than about the
> person we are angry with.

Instead, if we've decided to express our anger respectfully, we're more likely to say to the person who bumped into us, "Whoa! That took the wind out of me. Please watch your step." And to the person who showed up late, we might say, "I'm feeling annoyed and stressed because I've been holding dinner for you. I'm glad you're here, though, so let's get started."

As you grow out of your own EN, you'll discover that you'll get angry much less often. As your wounds heal, you won't get triggered as often, and you won't take what others do so personally. When you do get angry, you'll get over it far more quickly. You'll usually express the anger simply, directly, and respectfully—and then be done with it. And you won't use anger to distract yourself from feeling other, deeper emotions.

It's not wrong to feel or express anger. Anger only causes a problem when we hang onto it, stoke it, or express it disrespectfully. If we can explore it with curiosity, pay attention to what it is telling us, and then take positive action, we have used our anger wisely and well.

Anger always lets you know that something is wrong. Perhaps someone is treating you disrespectfully. Maybe you're hurting. Maybe you're temporarily caught in EN. When you feel anger rising up, it's important to notice it and, for a short time, simply observe it. Then decide what isn't right and take action to address the issue. This will get you better results than perpetuating the anger—or using it to distract yourself from what you feel beneath that anger.

## FEAR

Fear is an especially effective distractor. It can quickly and effectively remove us from almost any other feeling we don't want to deal with, by taking us out of our heart and into thought. The combination of fear, shame, and the five myths form the foundation of most of our EN.

All creatures, except for the very simplest ones, are born with an innate sense of fear. This fear is profoundly useful: it has kept our species alive for thousands of years. However, this fear is the fear of death and physical harm, and it typically only arises in the face of real or potential danger.

In contrast, when we use fear as a distractor, it is instead a fear of being

- rejected;
- inadequate or second rate;
- bad or wrong;
- unlikable or unlovable;

- not in control;
- embarrassed;
- alone;
- unattractive;
- stupid;
- judged (and, usually, disapproved of);
- looked down upon.

We need our fear to protect us and warn us of possible emotional or physical harm. However, fear is only useful for a few moments at a time. When we are not in some kind of real or possible danger, fear distracts us from the rest of our emotional life. It blocks us from feeling what else is really going on for us emotionally. It keeps us from feeling the pain of our EN.

When we stay in fear, we stop listening to our own heart and go off into our thoughts about what could happen. Fear has a way of taking over if we are not paying attention. It replaces our ordinary day-to-day, moment-by-moment faith that all will be well.

> When we are not in some kind of real or possible danger, fear distracts us from the rest of our emotional life.

Fear encourages us to mentally compose scenarios of doom. If we take these too seriously, these can create still more fear. If this becomes a habit, and the process continues looping back on itself, over time it can lead to anxiety, depression, or both.

## ARLEN

Arlen's girlfriend recently broke up with him. He fears he will never have another romantic relationship and spends hour after hour analyzing their breakup and becoming more and more frightened that he will go through life alone.

By focusing on his fear, Arlen doesn't have to deal with his other feelings: loneliness, hurt, embarrassment, and powerlessness. With his heart closed to his real feelings and distracted by his thoughts and his fear, he is not yet able to grieve—or to move through his grief to the relief just beyond it. Nor is he able to take care of himself and address any of his own needs.

## ATTEMPTING TO PLEASE OTHER PEOPLE

We've already looked at how the myths and principles of EN encourage us to compulsively try to please others. Now let's look at another aspect of people pleasing: how we use it as a major distractor.

In trying to please others, we turn our attention away from our own hearts, needs, and feelings. As we focus on what others want, we distract ourselves from the pain of not counting or being important, and our fear of being rejected.

### RENÉ AND DIANA

René, who is a mail carrier, comes home from work with a very sore foot. He looks forward to removing his shoes and massaging his foot with oil as soon as he has kissed his wife, Diana, hello.

When he gets inside, however, he sees immediately that Diana is in a bad mood. She is stomping around the kitchen and muttering to herself while fixing dinner. Uncomfortable with her anger and afraid she'll take it out on him, René quickly starts setting the table. He ignores the pain in his foot and his disappointment in coming home to his wife's anger. Instead, he asks Diana cheerfully, "How else can I help?"

She turns to him, holding an egg in each hand, and watches him for a few seconds. Then she says, "You can invent a time machine so we can start this crappy day over again." As she turns back toward the stove, she adds, "And why the hell are you limping?"

## VICTIM ENERGY

Victim energy distracts us in in three ways: First, our anger over being a victim distracts us from our deeper emotions; second, the stories we write in our head about being a victim can themselves be profound distractors; and third, because victim energy is pervasive in our society, and because it is usually socially acceptable to tell our stories of woe, we can readily share our victim energy with others. And when we do, we will often be rewarded for it with attention, sympathy, and (sometimes) empathy. Meanwhile, we distract ourselves from the very emotions we most need to feel if we are to heal.

### ANYA AND PARVIZ

Parviz and Anya came to see me because they were both unhappy in their marriage. It quickly became clear that Parviz struggled with a great deal of insecurity, the result of being seriously and repeatedly physically abused as a child. He almost constantly asked for Anya to tell him that she loved him. He also became demanding and critical when she disagreed with him or didn't do what he asked of her. Sometimes he would also accuse her of not loving or caring about him.

In our third session, Anya said to me, "Whenever Parviz and I have a conflict, he imagines I'm going to leave him. Then he pouts, or won't talk to me for days, or leaves the house for hours and won't answer my calls or texts. He makes up these crazy stories in his head about my running off. The longer he's gone, the longer and stranger the stories get. I reassure him, yet nothing I say or do ever seems to help."

Anya felt hopeless. She was stuck in Myth 1. She felt responsible for how Parviz felt and tried to fix his insecurities. Of course, nothing she did worked. How could it? Parviz's fears and insecurities were about himself, not about Anya. She started to become very tired of her husband not believing her, and she began to believe that things would never improve.

Anya had begun to create her own mental victim story in which she tried harder and harder, yet was never believed. She had begun to think that she might as well end the relationship. She also knew that the moment she did, Parviz would say, "I was right all along. You've been planning to leave me."

Parviz's victim stories distracted him from his shame, his sense of inadequacy, and his fear of being unlovable and unlikable. Anya's victim story prevented her from feeling her own sense of inadequacy (from not fulfilling Myth 1), as well as her powerlessness, fear, hurt, and discouragement.

Things did not improve until both Parviz and Anya began to examine the painful emotions beneath their mental victim stories and started the painful and necessary work of healing their EN.

## Willingness

Our distractors prevent us from having to experience many of our feelings. They also prevent us from having to experience our discomfort *about* those feelings.

Healing begins when we willingly walk into our emotions, and our discomfort about them, and stay with all the feelings long enough to name them and then work with them.

# MARGE

Marge, who is in her seventies, has had severe hip pain for over a year. She can only take three steps without needing to stop and rest. She is afraid of the surgery that could heal her hip, as well as the months of recovery and physical therapy that will be required afterward. So she has put off the surgery for several years.

Some of her friends had that same hip surgery, and Marge can see how much better they walk and how much more energy they have. Marge also sees how painful the recovery from the surgery was for them and how long required physical therapy lasted. Marge wants to avoid this pain and difficulty.

In avoiding that pain, however, Marge actually creates more pain for herself—and a disability as well. Eventually she reaches the point where every step is excruciating and she can no long walk unassisted.

This is when Marge makes the decision to walk into her fear and have the surgery. She realizes the pain she is experiencing is a destroying pain, bone grinding on bone. The pain from surgery and physical therapy, however, will be a healing pain, one that will likely end in time.

Marge courageously makes an appointment for surgery.

The operation is successful. At first there is a great deal of pain, which Marge willingly accepts. She also completes all the required physical therapy.

As the weeks pass, she is able to do more and more, and the pain begins to lessen. After three months, she can walk around her house with nothing more than discomfort, and after six months she has healed fully. For many years afterward, her hip is free of pain.

Left unattended, our emotions are like Marge's hip. They can grind away at our confidence, our self-esteem, our internal strength, and our belief in ourselves. However, if we are willing to walk into the necessary pain of feeling and trusting our emotions, we can clean out the old wounds so they can heal thoroughly. Over time, we too will become free of our old pain.

........................................................................................................

## GRACE

Grace, a thirty-five-year-old woman, came to see me. She suffered from depression, generalized anxiety, and panic attacks. She reported being afraid of almost everything in her life, especially things involving her children. Because of this, she had become irritable and short-tempered with her family. She didn't like the person she had become.

After several weeks of therapy, she became willing to share a part of her life that she had kept locked away for eighteen years. Mustering up her courage, she told me of being raped at gunpoint when she was seventeen. Afterward, wearing only a T-shirt, she convinced her rapist to let her stop home to pick up some clean clothes before he brought her somewhere else. He agreed. She ran into her house as soon as the car stopped and told her boyfriend what had happened to her. He went outside and assaulted the rapist, who broke free and drove off.

About thirty minutes later, the rapist returned with four of his friends and threatened them both with guns. Her boyfriend was able to temporarily calm everyone down, and the men eventually left. Before they did, however, they vowed to return sometime soon. "We're not done with you yet," one of them said to her boyfriend.

Grace and her boyfriend moved the next day. She and her boyfriend decided not to report the crimes to the police and kept them secret from family and friends. For years afterward, Grace lived in fear that the rapist and his friends would find her.

Now, almost two decades later, she decided to keep the events secret no longer. She was willing to walk into the discomfort of reliving those experiences. First she told her story to me. Then, with courage and willingness, she once again walked into her pain and told her mother. Then she made the choice to tell her father, then her sister, then her friends. Each time she made this choice, her healing deepened. Her family's love and acceptance helped her grow stronger. Her fear and anxiety decreased each day.

Today Grace is far less anxious, much more confident in herself, less irritable at home, and happier with her life. It all began with her willingness and courage to walk into her discomfort. And it ended with a new life.

# 10

# How Everyday Narcissism Diminishes Our Relationships

"Tenderness and kindness are not signs of weakness and despair, but manifestations of strength and resolution."

*Khalil Gibran*

Because of our own and others' EN, creating and maintaining authentic relationships can be very difficult for us.

EN is the opposite of unconditional love—being loved just for being who we are, without qualification or judgment. As children, all of us desired this unconditional love. Sadly, because of our parents' EN, most of us didn't get it. As a result, most adults don't know what it feels like in our bodies to be loved unconditionally.

We walk around hungering for this love—yet most of us are unsure just what it is, what it looks or feels like, how it can be acquired, or even if it *can* be acquired, rather than freely and spontaneously given and received. It's like walking around a large grocery store, knowing there is something in there that you need, yet having no idea what it is or how or where to find it. Because you've never experienced it, you don't even know if you'll recognize it when you see it. Yet you can't stop looking for it—whatever *it* is—because your body yearns for it and recognizes its absence.

Because we are steeped in EN, we also don't know how to love *ourselves* unconditionally. We don't know how to love others unconditionally, either. In her book *Prisoners of Childhood*, Alice Miller describes our dilemma this way:

> . . . a little reflection soon shows how inconceivable it is really to love others (not merely to need them), if one cannot love oneself as one really is. And how could a person do that if, from the very beginning, he has had no chance to experience his true feelings and to learn to know himself? . . . How can you love something you do not know, something that has never been loved?

We yearn, hope, and look for someone who will love us for who we really are. Yet our attempts to connect with others take a very different trajectory: we reach out with a false self to other false selves. *Because of our EN, our very attempts to get what we most want get in the way of our finding it.*

When we live out of our EN, we unconsciously (and sometimes consciously) try to train everyone we meet to take care of us and meet all our needs—to do and be and say exactly what we want, nearly all the time. While this is especially true of our family members, it is usually also true of our coworkers, our neighbors, our dry cleaner, our car mechanic, servers in restaurants, baristas in coffee shops, strangers we meet on the street, and more or less everyone else we encounter.

As part of this training, we may try to manipulate or micromanage everyone. We may point out what they need to do differently or how they need to change. We may become critical or angry or dismissive when they fail to perfectly oblige us.

Unconsciously, we hope that if others consistently take care of us and meet our needs, then we will finally feel safe, and our wounds will be healed. The reality, of course, is just the opposite: the more we get people to bend to our will, the more we hunger for them to bend to our will in the future. At the same time, they are likely to become more resentful and noncompliant.

Because of our EN, we may also believe that if someone truly cares about us, they will magically read our mind, know exactly what we want, and then do it—thus making us, at last, feel safe and happy. If they don't intuit and do exactly what we want, we then conclude that they must not really care about us. Meanwhile, we ignore this important truth: *even as we pull one string after another to get others to care for us, we do little to care for or love ourselves.*

In order to begin to heal, we need to let go of our EN and begin to create authentic relationships—first with ourselves, then with others. As you will discover, authentic relationships are the container for your healing.

# 11

# When Others Touch Our Wounds

*"The best and most beautiful things in the world cannot be seen, nor touched . . . but are felt in the heart."*

*Helen Keller*

Because of our and others' EN, most of us live our lives as the walking wounded. This is no mere metaphor. When we were children, most of us were repeatedly wounded by the people around us because of their own EN. Some of these emotional wounds remain in our bodies today, stored as trauma.

We subconsciously try to heal these wounds by getting others to take care of us. Yet this has precisely the opposite effect. Instead of healing us, our actions only deepen our wounds.

Because of EN, we have created a world in which nearly all of us have unhealed emotional wounds—and in which, through our

EN, we continue to wound each other in exactly the same ways, over and over.

We also wound each other accidentally. Think of a time when you said or did something innocuous, and suddenly the person you were with went ballistic on you. What likely happened? Without realizing it, you stepped on one of the person's EN wounds.

Now think of a time when someone said or did something that *they* felt was innocuous, and *you* suddenly went ballistic on *them*. They likely triggered one of your own EN wounds.

Here are some common over-the-top things people do when their EN wounds get triggered:

- Become very angry.
- Cry.
- Blame the other person for how miserable their life is, all the problems they have, etc.
- Blame the other person for being rude, thoughtless, uncaring, mean-spirited, heartless, stupid, etc.
- Blame themselves—e.g., "I knew I shouldn't have let someone like you drive me to work. I'm such a fool."
- Pout.
- Seethe.
- Become quiet and withdrawn.
- Refuse to speak or make eye contact.
- Pretend not to hear.
- Yell.
- Become physically violent.

## CLARISSA AND DREW

Let's consider an ordinary couple, Clarissa and Drew. When Drew inadvertently steps on one of Clarissa's EN wounds, she usually responds in one of the ways listed earlier. That response in turn may trigger one of Drew's EN wounds.

Drew then typically responds by *deliberately* poking another of Clarissa's EN wounds. The interaction soon escalates into a shouting match, or passive-aggressive, quiet seething—or, occasionally, physical violence.

Yet, even as the conflict escalates, neither person has a clue about what is happening or why their seemingly ordinary conversation quickly turns into something toxic. Each partner is also convinced the other is entirely to blame. In the end, nothing gets resolved, and both people are more wounded than ever.

When a couple first comes to me for therapy, I usually ask them what made them decide to seek couple's counseling. Most tell me, with some embarrassment, that they had a huge fight over "something stupid, something so little." Almost always, it turns out that the fight was not actually about the "something." *It was about triggering each other's unhealed childhood wounds.* Both people were operating from their EN, and each was trying desperately to be heard, or cared for, or loved, or valued. Yet each one instead stepped repeatedly on the other's old wounds.

In such cases, the solution is not just better communication techniques. *It is for each person to look at, recognize, and name their own wounds.* This means fully feeling and naming their emotions; recognizing and naming any needs that are not getting met; and then finding a way to meet each of those needs on their own.

Each person can then learn how to care for themselves, and then others, in a loving way. *This* is what will enable both partners to fully heal their EN, and live happier, more satisfying lives—separately and together.

## Observing Your Emotions

When someone has a sudden, over-the-top negative reaction to you, keep in mind their reaction is not about you at all, even though your own EN might tell you otherwise. One of their own childhood wounds was triggered. And whenever *you* have a big, sudden negative reaction to someone, it usually means that one of your own EN wounds from childhood was triggered.

It's also important to remember that when one of your own childhood wounds does get triggered, your thought process—your prefontal cortex—has largely shut down. Your amygdala—the part of your brain responsible for the fight, flight, or freeze response—is temporarily in charge.

In the future, whenever you have an abrupt, extreme reaction, please consider it a gift because it is the best and easiest way for you to recognize one of your own childhood wounds. Once you do recognize it as such, you can identify it, learn from it, and begin to heal it.

## Stepping into Healing

The first step in healing your EN wounds is understanding and accepting this simple, powerful principle: *No one else can heal your wounds for you. You must heal them yourself.*

> As you heal your childhood wounds and release yourself from the bondage of EN, you will begin to experience what unconditional love feels like.

Accepting this may hurt for a time. The good news, though, is that the pain will be temporary—and it will be far less painful than the accumulated, ongoing pain of not healing.

The even better news is that this healing is entirely possible. Many, many people have done it successfully and are now living fuller, more connected, more joyful lives as a result. I invite you to join them.

As you heal your childhood wounds and release yourself from the bondage of EN, you will begin to experience what unconditional love feels like. Day by day, you will learn how to fully love yourself for who you genuinely are. In the process, you will also develop the capacity to love others for who *they* genuinely are.

## HEALING ACTIVITY #16

### Address Your Needs

Most of the emotional wounds we carry with us from childhood are the result of needs that did not get met, often repeatedly. Each of these wounds can easily get triggered when a real-time event mirrors or reminds us of that unmet need from long ago. An important step in healing these wounds is coming to know and name each of these unmet needs. Please do the following:

**Within the next few days:**

1. Spend a few minutes reviewing the list of essential human needs, which appears immediately after this activity and at the end of this book.

2. In your healing notebook, write a list of all the needs that you remember not getting fulfilled in your childhood.

3. If there are any needs that *repeatedly* did not get met, circle these.

**In the weeks and months to come:**

1. Every two months, review your list and compare it to the list of essential human needs. If you recognize any other unmet needs, add them to your list.

2. Whenever you have an over-the-top reaction, remind yourself that it stems from an old, unhealed wound that has been triggered. Beneath this wound is a need that wasn't met in your childhood.

3. As soon as you can, stop whatever you are doing—shouting, pouting, blaming the other person, blaming yourself, planning your revenge, etc.

4. It may help to temporarily disengage. Say, "Give me a few moments to calm down," or "Let me go to the

bathroom; I'll be right back." Take a few deep breaths, or a walk around the block.

5. Remind yourself that the most important thing you can do is *not* teach the other person a lesson, or try to fix them or change them, or get them to take care of you. Instead, calmly, and with a lot of compassion, investigate your own wound.

6. As soon as you reasonably can, turn to the list of feelings at the end of this book. Reflect on your recent, over-the-top reaction, and write a list of all the feelings you experienced in connection with it.

7. Then turn to the list of needs you compiled in your healing notebook. Look through this list and name the needs you felt were not being met in that moment. These needs will reveal or point to old, unhealed wounds.

8. Remember that learning to identify and name a need that has not been met takes time and practice. Be patient with yourself. Over time, with the help of the list of needs, you will learn to do this.

9. Write a list of several specific things you can do to meet some or all of those needs yourself, rather than try to get others to meet them for you. As you create this list, don't evaluate any idea yet, or label it as good or bad. That will get in the way of your creative process. Write down all your ideas now; you'll have a chance to evaluate them later, once the list is complete. (This step may be painful and challenging the first few times. You may be used to figuring out what you want other people to do to make you feel better—and much less familiar with finding ways to meet your needs on your own.)

10. Once you're done making the list, review it carefully and decide which option is likely to work best for you.

11. Take action. Do the specific thing you chose. In this process, you take responsibility for meeting your need.

12. If the option you selected didn't work, try a different one. Repeat as necessary.

Once you have practiced this healing activity at least half a dozen times, expand your awareness to include any situation in which you feel unexpected pain, discomfort, or uneasiness. Review your list of unmet needs to see which one(s) the situation reflects or points to.

## Essential Human Needs

| | |
|---|---|
| Being | Clothing |
| – believed | Connection |
| – believed in | Emotional safety |
| – comforted | Emotional security |
| – counted | Kindness |
| – heard | Nourishment |
| – liked | Physical safety |
| – loved | Physical security |
| – taken seriously | Respect |
| – trusted | Shelter |
| – valued | Trust |
| Belonging | Unconditional acceptance |
| Caring | Unconditional love |

The following story is an example of how this process works.

## MICHAEL AND GAYLE

When Michael and Gayle first came to see me, each was very annoyed with the other, for multiple reasons. One of these had to do with time.

Being on time was very important to Michael. He believed that being late was disrespectful and rude. Gayle, however, was consistently late. When they went places together, they often ended up being late—and angry with each other. Both were stuck in Myth 2.

After going through this experience many times, Michael decided it was time for him to take care of his own feelings and needs.

I helped Michael to learn and practice the steps described earlier in this chapter. Over time, he was able to identify and name his emotions around Gayle's lateness: hurt, embarrassment, and powerlessness.

Then he identified his biggest unmet needs: his need for respect and his need for caring. From Michael's viewpoint, Gayle didn't respect his need to be on time and didn't care about him enough to seriously consider what he wanted. She simply did what she pleased.

Michael listed several options for how he could meet these needs *himself* in the future:

1. Accept Gayle's routine tardiness and plan to be late as well.

2. Apologize to his hosts and blame Gayle each time.

3. Go to events separately and meet Gayle there.

4. Not go to events at all and blame Gayle.

5. Let Gayle know the time he wants to leave, and tell her that if she is not ready by then, he will leave and meet her at the event.

6.  Tell Gayle how he feels when they are late—
    discounted, hurt, embarrassed, powerless,
    disrespected, and angry—and explain to her that
    he needs her to respect and care about him and his
    desire to be on time.

7.  Regularly tell Gayle that they need to arrive one hour
    earlier than they actually do.

Michael decided to start with option six. If things *didn't*
change, he would then try option five.

At first, things *didn't* change. Michael's request for Gayle to
care about his feelings and needs hadn't worked previously,
and it didn't work this time. He made the request simply and
straightforwardly, without anger, and he hoped that would
make a difference, yet it didn't. (Asking for what you want
from someone else is always fine. However, it's important
that you not *expect* to get what you ask for.)

Then Michael chose option five. At first he was frightened
to try this option because Myths 1, 3, and 5 echoed in his
brain, telling him that his choice would lead to all kinds of
trouble. He tried it anyway—and it worked beautifully. As
before, Gayle didn't change. However, Michael did.

Michael ended up getting to his sister's birthday party on
time, half an hour before Gayle—who was late, as usual.
What made the evening different was that both of them
greatly enjoyed it, and neither felt anger or resentment
toward the other.

Since then, Michael and Gayle have continued to follow
option five, and it has continued to work for both of them.

---

Dealing with your own unmet needs will often require you to
look both backward and forward. You can begin by looking backward
at a recent (or not-so-recent) difficulty. Because most difficulties
follow patterns, revisiting one from your past can help you to see

what choice you made, why you made it, and what other choices you had at the time. You can then use this awareness to plan how you will take care of yourself in the future, if a similar situation arises.

As you will discover, taking care of yourself will become a habit—a very healthy habit. This will replace the old EN habits of trying to take care of others and trying to get them to take care of you. The more you take care of yourself, the better you will feel, the more and faster you will heal, and the more joy and serenity you will experience in your life.

There is one other key aspect to this shift: taking care of others and trying to control them often doesn't work. Yet taking care of yourself usually does. As you practice self-care, this will become increasingly clear.

Which of the following is more likely to work, and which is easier to make happen?

- Taking out your trash or trying to get your neighbors to take out theirs.

- Making a sandwich or trying to convince your partner to make one for you.

- Taking a hired car to the airport or finding someone to drive you.

This is why it's so essential, and so helpful, to make self-care a habit. It's a far saner, less stressful, and more rewarding habit than trying to control everyone and everything else.

# 12

# Creating a Healing Environment

The process of healing from EN can feel scary, uncomfortable, and perhaps even terrifying at first, because it requires us to do things very differently from what we are used to. These activities sometimes feel like they threaten our sense of belonging and being loved.

In fact, however, they do the opposite: they challenge the things we've done that haven't worked. They give us an opportunity to at last open our heart, love ourselves and others more fully, and be loved by them for who we are—not whom we imagine they want us to be.

To help support this healing process, you can create your own ideal healing environment through three moment-by-moment practices:

- Live in present time.
- Stop the story you're writing in your head.
- Nonattachment.

## Live in Present Time

Mentally and emotionally, most of us spend much of our time away from the present. We are often busy thinking about the future, and most of what we imagine or anticipate is scary or painful. Yet it is simply not real.

Instead, we can live in the moment—the only time we can really do anything about it, and the only time in which we have the power to make choices.

When you live in present time, you can check in with yourself by asking yourself these questions:

- *Am I okay right now?* (If so, simply stay in the present.)
- *Is there anything else I can or need to do right now to improve things? If so, what is my next task or step?* (Then take that step. If nothing needs to be done, simply return to present time.)

## Stop the Story You're Writing in Your Head

Our minds spend a great deal of time writing detailed stories about what might happen. While some of these are pleasant fantasies, most of them are based on our fears. Some of us are particularly good at this.

This story-writing process is both natural and unavoidable. What we *can* avoid, however, is taking these stories seriously.

Remember Marcia, the woman who wrote a story in her head about being alone on Christmas? On her way to work, while enjoying a beautiful fall day, she made herself cry by just making up a mental story of loneliness.

When you catch yourself writing a story in your head, smile, acknowledge what you're doing, and then mentally stop the story. If the story created fear, anger, or sadness, remind yourself that nothing has actually happened. All you did was write a mental story that frightened or angered or saddened you.

Once you realize what you are doing, come back to the present. Pay attention to where you are right now—in your car, at your job, walking the dog, eating. Look at what is around you; feel your way back into your body; note any sounds, smells, tastes, or other sensations. Get back into what is actually going on. Then enjoy this moment of freedom from writing stories in your head and the misery they can create. When you're able to catch and stop this story writing, you will be amazed how much better life feels.

## Nonattachment

Most of us have spent our lives stuck in EN, doing our utmost to control the people and events around us—all so we can be liked, loved, and accepted. As we've learned, though, this simply doesn't work.

Nonattachment may be the most difficult tool to learn because most of us live in some form of attachment. We're attached to the car we drive, or how much money we make, or the home or neighborhood we live in.

Many of us even come to believe that the things we're attached to define who we are. (One of the central tenets of Buddhism is that such a view of who we are is a delusion.) Another common form of attachment involves wanting particular outcomes to occur: getting a particular job, having the perfect party, getting into our preferred college.

Often we're so attached to a particular person or dream or outcome that we choose to overlook some clear warning signs. Many people who come into my therapy office are unhappy in their marriages. Often they begin by telling me about their partner's drinking, anger, spending, criticizing, or some other negative trait. I ask them if they saw any warning signs of this behavior while they were dating, or if their own inner wisdom had suggested at the time that there might be problems. Usually the answer is yes. However, they were so attached to the person, or to getting married, that they chose to ignore the warnings. Now they are living with the visible, predictable problems.

Often when we need to make a decision, we can become so attached to a particular choice that we ignore our own inner wisdom, or information from external sources, that would redirect us if only we paid attention to it. This can involve something large and important, such as choosing a partner, buying a house, or taking a new job; it can also involve something as common and everyday as speaking your truth, caring for yourself, or saying no.

Nonattachment is letting go of trying to control the outcome, or the direction things may take. This goes against all the myths and principles of EN, which teach us that we can and must control all outcomes, so others will be happy, like us, and make us happy, too.

In nonattachment, you live with letting things unfold as they may, trusting that you will be guided and, if you pay attention, it will all be well. Yet most of us have spent our lives in EN, doing just the opposite, trying to control things—and failing, over and over, because actually there is not much in life we can genuinely control.

Letting go of this imaginary control is challenging and scary at first. It also means learning to approach your choices in a different way. Instead of simply trying to wrest control of the situation, you often need to research other options, seek advice, and be realistic about the possible consequences of any choice you make. You also need to accept your disappointment if you are guided in a different or unexpected direction, or if things don't go the way you hoped.

In nonattachment, you learn to accept and live into unexpected and undesired outcomes. Frequently, though, to your surprise, those outcomes present you with new possibilities and choices. You let things unfold, trusting that if you are present, you will get the guidance you need. You do your best in each situation, while letting go of the outcome. You engage fully with what is happening without trying to control it and make it bend to your will. You stay as present as you can with what is happening in each moment—including your emotions, your impulses, and the events unfolding around you. You understand, deep in your body and heart, that this way of living is essential to your happiness.

Nonattachment is very different from passivity. You don't refuse to act. You continue to make decisions and take action. However, you let yourself be guided by your wisdom instead of desperately trying to control outcomes.

As you practice nonattachment, you don't expect everyone (or anyone) else to take care of you. Instead, you take care of yourself as best you can. You listen to the wisdom within you and trust it. You also stay open to guidance from many other sources: your friends; something that stands out in a magazine article; something you notice on TV or a bumper sticker; or any of a thousand others. It might be as simple as *Put your book by your purse or you'll forget it tomorrow morning.*

Or it might be as important as *I don't like being around Harry's anger. He gets so angry so often. I'm starting to feel scared around him. If that doesn't change, I need to stop dating him. I love him with all my heart, yet his anger is starting to become a serious problem.*

This also means allowing yourself to be briefly disappointed when the guidance you receive isn't what you wanted to hear. Yet if it strikes you as correct or valuable, don't brush it away because it's not what you expected. Not listening to guidance that you know in your heart is important usually leads to unhappiness.

As you'll discover, when you listen and act on the guidance that feels right, you will be much happier in the long run, even if, for the moment, you are disappointed. You may not enjoy getting out of your warm, comfortable bed to put the book by your purse, yet you'll be glad in the morning that you have it with you. If you end up breaking up with your partner because of their anger, you'll naturally feel sad; however, not as sad as if you marry that person, and their anger turns into abuse.

Healing from EN is ultimately a spiritual act. When we live according to EN, we make it into a god: we follow its commands in the false hope that it will bring us safety, love, and acceptance. We eventually discover that it always fails us.

As we heal, we lose our faith in EN's lies, myths, and false promises. We replace it with faith in something genuine and true: full engagement with life itself.

Over time, we learn to trust that happiness and serenity are available to us. They are some of the natural results of no longer trying to control the world; instead, we let go and open to it. Many people describe this shift as connecting to a Higher Power.

The more you incorporate these practices—living in present time, stopping the stories in your head, and nonattachment—the more your fear will subside, and the more serenity, relief, and joy you will experience.

These three activities have the ability to radically change your life for the better. They will lead you back to your authentic self. And with practice, they will eventually become as natural as breathing.

# 13

# Everyday Forgiveness

"Forgiveness is letting go of the hope that
the past can be changed."

*Oprah Winfrey*

Most of us were taught the importance of forgiving others. We were told how much happier we would be if we forgave, yet no one really taught us *how* to forgive. In fact, others may have shamed us for not forgiving others—or not forgiving them quickly or easily enough. We may also have shamed ourselves for not being able to easily let go and forgive.

Meanwhile, our EN may create a variety of resentments and anger that we carry around with us. We feel betrayed, let down, and hurt. We repeatedly say to ourselves, in essence, *I routinely set aside my own wants and needs, and take care of the wants and needs of others.* (Myths 1, 3, and 4) *So why aren't other people caring for me?* (Myth 2) This anger and resentment make forgiveness impossible. And to stay angry, we have to keep writing our victim stories in our heads—our stories of how we were hurt, mistreated, betrayed, and so on. This takes up a great deal of time and energy.

As we heal our EN and live life from our authentic self, we will naturally begin to let go of our anger and resentment. At the same time, the urge to keep mentally writing our story of victimhood will slowly and steadily subside.

## Getting to Know Forgiveness

People frequently misunderstand what forgiveness is really about. So let's begin by looking at what it is not, so we can more readily explore what it is.

Forgiveness . . .

- is not about letting someone off the hook.
- does not mean you approve of the person's behavior.
- does not mean you have to like the person.
- is not something you do for the other person's benefit.
- is not a requirement or a "should."
- does not mean you agree with what the person said or did.
- does not require you to be vulnerable to the person.
- does not mean you have to be friends.
- is not an act of will.
- is not a plan or technique.
- is not about forgetting or ignoring the past.
- does not mean you don't hold the other person accountable.

Forgiveness *does* require us to have an open heart, to stay connected to ourselves, and to be connected with others. It arises naturally when our heart is open and we allow compassion to emerge.

Freedom is the natural outcome of forgiveness.

# UMA

In my office, Uma described to me a recurring memory she had had from the age of eight. She lay on her neighbor's lawn—hands behind her head, knees drawn up—and looked up into the cloudless blue sky. She noticed half a dozen birds high in the sky. They rarely flapped their wings; instead, they rode the air currents, tipping, diving, and changing direction. It looked wonderful to be so free, to soar.

While watching those birds, Uma hungered to feel that free. She decided that one day she would.

Later in life, Uma found herself tired of carrying around all the ancient, heavy anger she felt toward her mother. That's when she made an appointment with me.

In therapy, Uma learned that her anger at her mother was covering deep pain—the pain of her mother not seeing how precious she was, how sweet she was, how much she had to give.

Uma sat across from me in my office. For an hour, her tears flowed. Then she felt the pain leave her body. Soon it was replaced with a deep realization of her own sweetness and preciousness. She no longer needed her anger at her mother to distract her from that pain.

Uma also began to see her mother's pain as well. For the first time, she understood in her body that her mother was never good enough for grandma. She understood that her mother's inability to see Uma's preciousness was entirely her mother's issue, her own EN.

Soon afterward, forgiveness and compassion arose naturally. Uma's anger at her mother blew away like smoke in the wind, and she felt tremendous freedom, lightheartedness, and giddiness. Then she remembered those birds above the neighbor's yard. She realized that she was now soaring, ready to move on with her life in a new way.

This same outcome—and the same freedom—are available to all of us. If we choose to heal from EN, our hearts will open, and we will naturally find freedom, forgiveness, compassion, and serenity.

## CARLA AND HARRIET

Carla and Harriet are next-door neighbors. Harriet does her best to be compassionate and friendly to everyone on her block. Carla, however, is an alcoholic who is often verbally abusive to the people who live nearby.

Harriet and Carla both own dogs. When Harriet first moved into the neighborhood, she hoped their shared interest in dogs would encourage Carla to be friendlier to her. Unfortunately, that didn't happen. Several times, Carla has said to her, "If your dog ever shows up on my property, I'm making two calls—one to the animal control people to cart your dog away, and one to the police to have you arrested."

One morning, Harriet lets her two Scottish terriers out into her fenced yard. She doesn't realize that, only a few moments earlier, Carla had let her spaniels out into her own yard. Within seconds, the dogs are a foot apart, on opposite sides of the shared fence, barking loudly and angrily at each other.

A minute later, Carla comes running out her back door, her face twisted in fury. "You bitch!" she screams at Harriet. "What the hell is wrong with you?"

Harriet hurries out her own backdoor. She waves at Carla and shouts back, "Sorry! I didn't realize your dogs were outside! I'll call my girls in. Heather! Beatrice! Come here!"

Harriet's dogs run to her. Carla's dogs run toward her, too, up to the fence. Then Carla leans over and shouts a stream of angry curses at Harriet.

Harriet starts to usher her dogs back inside. As she does, Carla shouts, "Don't bail on me, you whore! You come back here right now so I can tell you to your face what I think of you and your shitty dogs!"

Harriet takes a deep breath, steps inside, and closes and locks the door behind her. After giving each of her dogs a treat, she sits down and tells herself how grateful she is that she does not live a life like Carla's. She wishes Carla well and hopes that she will find serenity one day. Then Harriet gets on with her day.

Harriet is able to respond with forgiveness and compassion. Instead of making herself Carla's victim, she opens her heart to her—in circumstances that are private and protected.

## Forgiveness Is a Form of Self-Care

You forgive others as a part of your own healing. You forgive in order to put down that big bag of resentments, spread your wings, and live the life you want to live. You forgive in order to stay (or become) connected to your own heart.

For the same reasons, you can also forgive *yourself* and let go of your self-directed anger, shame, and blame. With forgiveness comes peace and the opportunity to live in your authentic self.

What sentence about forgiveness is most often repeated and quoted? Jesus's prayer on the cross: "Father, forgive them, for they know not what they do."

> With forgiveness comes peace and the opportunity to live in your authentic self.

Why does this quote deeply affect so many of us, including people who aren't Christians? Perhaps it is because, even in his dying moments, Jesus stayed connected to his heart. He remained caring and compassionate to everyone around him, even the people who were harming him.

## How Forgiveness Emerges

Over time, as you heal your EN, you will discover that forgiveness—both for yourself and for others—naturally emerges and grows inside you. In particular, the healing activity you began practicing in Chapter Eight, "Love the Child Inside You," can encourage your heart to open and prepare it to forgive. Please continue to practice this activity daily, even if only for a minute or two.

At times, however, you may still feel caught in old anger or resentment toward others, based on what they did weeks, months, or years ago. When this anger or resentment bubbles up, a similar activity can help you feel it, let go of it, and open a space for forgiveness to grow.

---

## HEALING ACTIVITY #17

### Prepare Your Heart to Forgive

- Find a calm, private place where you can sit quietly for a few minutes. Get settled.

- Think of the person you are angry with, or resentful toward, as well as the specific event or events behind your anger or resentment.

- Now, gently, feel your way into the emotions *beneath* the anger or resentment. These might include grief, or disappointment, or confusion, or hurt, or something else entirely. For the moment, just notice them, acknowledge them, name them, and sit with them as they arise.

- Remind yourself that when others have harmed you, their actions stemmed from *their* pain and struggles.

- Also remind yourself that, although the myths and principles of EN blame *you* for their actions, those myths and principles are all false. When other people harm you, *they* are responsible for what they've done, not you.

- Consider the possibility that the person did not intend to hurt you or simply made an honest mistake. If this seems likely, or strongly possible, remind yourself that you, too, make honest mistakes and at times have hurt others without intending to—and would want to be forgiven.

- Remember compassion. Imagine the other person's life: their struggles, their limitations, their difficulties, their sources of pain, what it must be and feel like to be them.

- Ask yourself if you would like to have the same struggles and difficulties they do. If not, be grateful that you don't, and that you are able to choose to do your own life differently.

- Accept the person for who they are, without judgment. Then decide whether and how much you want that person to remain in your life.

- Going forward, set clear boundaries with this person that support your decision and keep you safe.

You're probably familiar with this old saying: *To err is human; to forgive, divine.* This is just another myth. Forgiveness is *not* merely divine; it is also deeply and profoundly human.

A few years ago, I attended a talk by a survivor of Theresienstadt, a Nazi concentration camp in World War II that served as a transit point for people en route to Auschwitz. Of the 15,000 children who entered the camp, ninety-three survived. The speaker was one of those ninety-three.

This survivor, who was then in his eighties, shared some of his experiences in the camp. At the end of his speech he told of reuniting a few years earlier with a man he had known in the camp. He asked that man how he was feeling now. His fellow survivor began by shouting, "I hate those Nazis! I hate those Nazis!"

The speaker's response to his fellow survivor was, "I'm sorry to hear that. It means they still have you imprisoned."

This aging man had forgiven the Nazis—not because they deserved it, or because so much time had passed. He forgave them because he had chosen to open his heart, to go beyond his anger and resentments. He chose to no longer be imprisoned by his past, his emotions, or the suffering he endured. After all the trauma he had experienced, he was able to forgive—and find his authentic self.

If he could do this, then you too can heal your own wounds and live from your own authentic self, free of the myths and shackles of EN.

# 14

# Everyday Healing

"Don't ask what the world needs. Ask what makes
you come alive, and go do it. Because what the
world needs is people who have come alive."

*Howard Thurman*

Creating the life you want takes courage, determination, and a
commitment to heal and change. It also requires a willingness to look
inward for answers instead of looking to others to make you happy.

---

## HEALING ACTIVITY #18

---

### Integrate What You Have Learned into Your Life

Here's a quick review of the many things you can do, day by
day, to heal your EN:

- Notice the multiple ways and forms in which the five myths of EN permeate your life and the lives of others around you.

- When you feel one of the myths arising inside you, recognize it, name it, and let go of it. Return to your authentic self.

- Set clear boundaries with others, and be clear with yourself about what those boundaries are.

- Speak your truth with honesty and kindness.

- Recognize each of your defenses and the impulse to use one. Then let go of it.

- Notice your shame when it arises, and simply sit with it and feel it. Then use the tools in this book to help heal the shame.

- Recognize and identify an old wound whenever it gets triggered.

- Over time, become familiar with the kinds of words, thoughts, and events that trigger these wounds.

- Become familiar with your needs that weren't met.

- Regularly find multiple ways to fulfill your needs on your own.

- Test out various strategies for fulfilling each need until you find one that works.

- Love and care for yourself.

You cannot heal in isolation. It will be very helpful if you have (or can find) a friend—or, better, three or four friends—with whom you can be authentic. Let them see the real you; share your successes and struggles with them; care for them; and, most of all, let them care for you. (This might feel quite uncomfortable at first.) The more you show a real friend your authentic self, the more opportunities you create for real connection, support, caring, and love.

Day by day, as you heal your everyday narcissism, you will discover more confidence, more power, and more joy.

> The more you show a real friend your authentic
> self, the more opportunities you create for real
> connection, support, caring, and love.

## Looking Back and Forward

For a moment, let's consider what you've gained, and will continue to gain, from your process of healing:

- Freedom from the pain and imprisonment of past events.
- Freedom from the endless repetition of resentful thoughts.
- Freedom from shame.
- Freedom from the myths, principles, and lies of EN.
- Freedom to live in the present, with all its possibilities, rather than in the past, with all its old hurts.
- Freedom to move toward the life you most want to live.

## Some Final Words of Hope

Everyday narcissism is as common as sadness and happiness. Yet we all need to remember that EN is not an inherent part of being human. *It is something each of us learned.* Because we learned it, we can unlearn it as well. You have already begun this process.

You have also learned new skills for healing your wounds and taking charge of your life. I encourage you to continue practicing these—encounter by encounter, day by day—until they become natural parts of your life.

EN is everywhere in our culture. Now that you have become aware of it, you will see it at work, at family gatherings, in places of worship, in schools, at restaurants, in the media—*everywhere.* (One clue: whenever you hear gossip, whining, or complaining, you're probably observing someone reacting from their EN.)

Although EN pervades our lives, it need not control them. As you heal your own EN, your life will improve. You will not feel hurt as often. And when you *are* hurt, it will be more like a scratch than a knife wound. You will see that the way people treat you is mostly about them and their choices, not you.

You'll feel much less stress, fear, and emotional pain. You'll be more in control of what goes on in your life. You'll feel both more powerful and more serene.

Best of all, the improvement won't end with your own life. As you heal your own EN, the world will become a kinder, more respectful, more loving, and more honest place. One person and one action at a time, your healing will change the world for the better.

# Recommended Resources

*The Body Keeps the Score* by Bessel van der Kolk (book)

*The Drama of the Gifted Child* by Alice Miller (book)

*Getting Unstuck* by Pema Chödrön (audio)

*The Power of Now* by Eckhart Tolle (book)

*Prisoners of Childhood* by Alice Miller (book)

*The Ultimate Happiness Prescription: 7 Keys to Joy and Enlightenment* by Deepak Chopra (book)

## The False Principles Behind Everyday Narcissism

1. I am responsible for how other people feel and behave. Therefore, I experience myself as all-powerful.

2. I am responsible for how others act toward *me*. Therefore, I once again experience myself as all-powerful.

3. Other people are responsible for how *I* feel and behave—and are supposed to make me feel safe, happy, and okay. Therefore, I am the center of the universe.

# FEELINGS

| | | |
|---|---|---|
| Abandoned | Cared for | Discounted |
| Affectionate | Carefree | Discouraged |
| Affirmed | Certain | Disempowered |
| Afraid | Charmed | Disgruntled |
| Alarmed | Cheated | Disgusted |
| Alive | Cheerful | Dismissive |
| Alone | Compassionate | Dissed |
| Ambivalent | Concerned | Distant |
| Angry | Confident | Distraught |
| Anxious | Conflicted | Distressed |
| Appalled | Confused | Distrustful |
| Appreciated | Constricted | Disturbed |
| Appreciative | Content | Dominated |
| Apprehensive | Controlled | Doubtful |
| Aroused | Crappy | Dumb |
| Ashamed | Crazy | Eager |
| Bad | Crushed | Elated |
| Bashful | Curious | Embarrassed |
| Betrayed | Deceived | Emboldened |
| Bewildered | Defeated | Empathetic |
| Blessed | Defensive | Empowered |
| Blue | Delighted | Empty |
| Bored | Demeaned | Encouraged |
| Bound | Depressed | Energetic |
| Brave | Despairing | Energized |
| Burdened | Desperate | Enervated |
| Buzzed | Devastated | Entitled |
| Calm | Diminished | Envious |
| Capable | Disappointed | Excited |

| | | |
|---|---|---|
| Exhausted | Ignored | Numb |
| Fearful | Impatient | Open |
| Fearless | Imposed upon | Oppressed |
| Firm | Impotent | Panicky |
| Flushed | Inadequate | Patient |
| Flustered | Incapable | Passionate |
| Fortunate | Inept | Peaceful |
| Frantic | Inferior | Pleased |
| Frenetic | Inspired | Powerful |
| Frightened | Intimidated | Powerless |
| Gay | Invisible | Pressured |
| Generous | Isolated | Proud |
| Giddy | Jealous | Put upon |
| Glad | Joyful | Rejected |
| Grateful | Jubilant | Relaxed |
| Grief-stricken | Jumpy | Released |
| Guilty | Kind | Relieved |
| Happy | Left out | Remorseful |
| Healthy | Listless | Rested |
| Held back | Lonely | Restless |
| Helpful | Lost | Reticent |
| Helpless | Loved | Revolted |
| Hesitant | Loving | Romantic |
| High | Melancholy | Run down |
| Honored | Miserable | Sad |
| Hopeful | Motivated | Safe |
| Hopeless | Mournful | Satisfied |
| Humble | Nauseated | Scared |
| Humiliated | Needed | Self-righteous |
| Hungry | Needy | Sexy |
| Hurt | Nervous | Shaky |

| | | |
|---|---|---|
| Shameful | Thankful | Unworthy |
| Shocked | Thrilled | Upset |
| Shy | Thwarted | Uptight |
| Sick | Tickled | Used |
| Sluggish | Tight | Violated |
| Somber | Tired | Vulnerable |
| Sorrowful | Tough | Wanted |
| Stifled | Trapped | Weak |
| Stressed | Troubled | Weary |
| Strong | Trusting | Weepy |
| Stuck | Uncertain | Wimpy |
| Stunned | Uneasy | Worn out |
| Stupid | Unappreciated | Worried |
| Suffocated | Unimportant | Worthy |
| Supported | Unloved | Wound up |
| Sympathetic | Unmotivated | Wrung out |
| Tense | Unsafe | |
| Terrified | Unsure | |

# ANGRY FEELINGS

| | | |
|---|---|---|
| Angry | Furious | Outraged |
| Annoyed | Hateful | Rageful |
| Cantankerous | Incensed | Resentful |
| Crabby | Indignant | Spiteful |
| Enraged | Indignant | Spiteful |
| Exasperated | Infuriated | Ticked off |
| Frustrated | Irritated | Vengeful |
| | Mad | |

# ESSENTIAL HUMAN NEEDS

| | |
|---|---|
| Being | Clothing |
| – believed | Connection |
| – believed in | Emotional safety |
| – comforted | Emotional security |
| – counted | Kindness |
| – heard | Nourishment |
| – liked | Physical safety |
| – loved | Physical security |
| – taken seriously | Respect |
| – trusted | Shelter |
| – valued | Trust |
| Belonging | Unconditional acceptance |
| Caring | Unconditional love |

# COMMON DISTRACTORS

Alcohol

Analyzing

Anger

Arrogance

Blame

Blogging

Children (caring for them, thinking about them, etc.)

Chores

Cleaning

Clubbing

Computer games

Complaining

Dating

Defiance

Denial

Drugs

Eating

Email

Entertaining (planning and hosting social events, etc.)

Exercising

Facebook

Fantasizing

Fear

Food (cooking, eating, collecting recipes, planning menus, etc.)

Gambling

Gardening

Googling

Gossiping

Hand work (crocheting, embroidery, needlepoint. Etc.)

Hobbies

Home maintenance and repair

Hosting or organizing events

Humor

Intellectualizing

Knitting

Judging others

Lying (either to others or to ourselves)

Meditation

Minimizing

Organizing (our home, our possessions, etc.)

Phoning

Playing sports

Pleasing others

Politics

Prayer

Pouting

Quilting

Rationalizing

Reading

Relationships

Religion

Revenge

Romance

School

Scrapbooking

Sex (having it, thinking about it,
and fantasizing about it)

Shopping

Smoking or other tobacco use

Social media

Socializing

Television

Texting

Twitter

Victim energy

Volunteering

Video games

Videos and movies

Watching sports

Weight loss or management

Women

Work

Writing mental stories

Yard work

# YOUR EN WALLET CARD

To help you recognize the myths of EN as you go about your day, carry this card with you in your purse or wallet.

---

## The Five Myths of Everyday Narcissism

1. We are responsible for—and have the power to control—how other people feel and behave.

2. Other people are responsible for—and have the power to control—the way we feel and behave.

3. The needs and wants of other people are more important than our own.

4. Following the rules is also more important than addressing our needs and feelings.

5. We are not lovable as we are; we can only become lovable through what we do and say.

Printed in the USA
CPSIA information can be obtained
at www.ICGtesting.com
JSHW022336140824
68134JS00019B/1526